More Praise for *Doing it*

"Isadora Alman tells it like it really is—no nastiness,
just the truth. Her sense of humor, her clarity, and her wisdom
cut through today's sexual confusion. If you want to be sure
you know what you're doing, read this book!"

—TINA TESSINA, PH.D., author of
The 10 Smartest Decisions A Woman Can Make After 40

"I recommend this valuable book for many reasons,
especially its emphasis on the importance of personal sharing,
clear communication, and on making nonjudgmental sex
information more widely available."

—MAGGI RUBENSTEIN, PH.D., Dean of Students Emeritus,
Institute for the Advanced Study of Human Sexuality; co-founder,
San Francisco Sex Information

Doing it

Doing **it**

Real People Having
Really Good **Sex**

I S A D O R A   A L M A N

CONARI PRESS
Berkeley, California

Conari Press books are distributed by Publishers Group West.

ISBN: 1-57324-520-8

Cover and Book Design: Suzanne Albertson
Author Photo: Lori Eanes

Library of Congress Cataloging-in-Publication Data

Alman, Isadora, 1940–
    Doing it : real people having really good sex / Isadora Alman.
        p.   cm.
    Includes index.
    ISBN 1-57324-520-8
  1. Sex. 2. Sex customs. I. Title.
HQ21 .A4524 2001
306.7—dc21
                                                    00-011385

Printed in Canada on recycled paper.

00 01 02 03   TC   10 9 8 7 6 5 4 3 2 1

Doing**it**

Introduction 1

1 The Single State 5

On Being Single 6
The Sweetie Search 11
Where to Go A-Sweetie-Hunting 19

2 The Dating Game 23

The Shopping Process 24
Turn-ons 27
Turn-offs 31
Friends and Lovers 33
Nice Guys 35
"I'll Call You" 37
Aha! Sex! 41

3 Coupling 45

On Relationships 46
Monogamy and Polyamory 52
Long-Distance Relationships 57

4 The Body 63

Getting Physical 64
Tastes 65
Smells 67
Body Hair 68
Menstruation 73

Birth Control 74

Lubricants 79

Sexually Transmitted Diseases 80

5 Solo Sex 83

On the Act of Masturbation 84

For Herself 84

For Himself 88

For Your Partner 94

6 Outercourse 97

Sex Play 98

Nipples and Breasts 107

Sex Talk 110

Sex Toys 112

7 Intercourse 115

The Old In and Out 116

Sexual Housekeeping 123

8 Oral Sex on a Woman 125

9 Oral Sex on a Man 135

10 Anal Play 149

11 Varieties 161

Two's Company, Three's a Party 162

Cross-Dressing 165

Anal and Vaginal Fisting 167

Voyeurism and Exhibitionism 170
Power Play 171
Outside the Box 176

12 Men   177

The Penis 178
Size and Shape 178
Cut or Uncut 185
Erections 187
Orgasms and Ejaculations 192

13 Women   197

Anatomy 198
Arousal 201
Orgasms 203
Ejaculation 208
Menopause 210

14 Relationship Middles and Endings   215

Keeping the Spark Alive 216
Libido 221
Meds and Drugs 224
When It's Over 227

Postscript 231
Index 233
About the Author 241

introduction

Since 1984 I have been writing a sex and relationship column called "Ask Isadora." Through the years I have been deluged, inundated, and often overwhelmed by mail, some typed on office stationary, some written in pencil on raggedly torn school paper. Some letters give me absolutely no clue as to the age, circumstances, or even the sex of the letter writer, and I answer as if sexual happiness questions and their answers can cross most lines of age, gender, and orientation, which, of course, they do. Some letter writers do identify themselves—"a thirty-four-year-old straight woman, married, in good shape"—even down to eye color, as if they supposed I'd have a different response for someone with brown eyes than I would for someone with blue. Those who sign their names rather than something like "Desperate in Detroit" invariably ask me not to print it, as if I might say, "This letter about her secret extramarital lesbian affair is from Betty Bumpety in Hartford."

The "Ask Isadora" column has appeared in several dozen alternative newspapers and magazines over the years, in many cities in three countries. There is no pattern to all the mail I have received, nothing that distinguishes the worries of readers in Toronto from those in Baltimore, nor, really, those of men from those of women. (Feel free to add to the load by writing me care of the *San Francisco Bay Guardian*, 520 Hampshire Street, San Francisco, CA 94110.) The letters just keep on coming in, and the woes occasioned by sex seem never-ending and remarkably repetitive.

Obviously I don't have all the answers, and often a different slant or more information could have enhanced the response I supplied in my brief column. So I receive a smaller, but still significant, amount of mail whose purpose is to continue the conversation, with me or with other letter writers: "Tell that lonely guy that he should take dance classes. It worked for me" or, "She might try smearing on unflavored yogurt and see if that helps." Because an individual's experience can include things mine doesn't, professionally or personally (like the recent how and where of purchasing and fitting a male chastity belt), I have frequently run Readers' Responses columns that contain the good ("What a great column!"), the bad ("Tell that guy to see a doctor ASAP"), and the ugly ("You Jezebel, you'll burn in hell!"). This kind of reader-to-reader exchange inspired the idea behind this book, which is not about my advice to readers but their advice to each other.

In 1996, eLine, a Web design firm, and I put online a version of the "Ask Isadora" column that was created to facilitate discussion among those interested in sex without requiring me in the middle. The website is *www.askisadora.com*. In the more than four years my Sexuality Forum (originally Advanced Birds & Bees) has been online in various formats, it alone has occasioned more than a million posts—questions, commentary, and/or responses.

The immediacy of the questions and answers in the Sexuality Forum is wonderful. (Not at all like the frequent months that elapse between the time someone mails me a letter and the time I *might* get to it in my washtub-sized mail basket; many never get answered.) At 9 P.M., after I have turned off my computer for the evening, someone might post a question about how to approach an attractive stranger. By 9 A.M. the next morning, when I again check into the site, there may be twenty or thirty suggestions from various people, plus an offshoot discussion or two on the trials and tribulations of being single ... and perhaps a few flirtatious comments aimed at other posters as well.

The tips in this book are gathered from both the column readers who wrote to their newspapers to carry on the conversation and posters to the Sexuality Forum who continue to create and maintain so many fascinating dialogues. In this book you will not be reading the opinions of one sex expert with whom you can agree or not or whose life experience you may or may not share. Instead, men and women of all ages and persuasions let you in on what they think are important details about sexual happiness. Often these details are secrets, in that there isn't anyone else in the writer's real life to whom they are willing to risk revealing these discoveries; so you will be the first to know, for instance, that twiddling nipples at a particular pace and direction will drive a woman wild ... or at least one woman, the writer or one in the writer's life.

I am often asked if a particular letter or post might be a put-on, or even if a large percentage might be. Sure, they *might* be. Occasional letters sound as if they were composed by a bunch of stoned college kids amusing themselves by stretching their imaginations and pulling my leg. I think you'll agree, though, that most of these responses have the ring of truth. I don't doubt that they are written by real people having real sex, and, often, really good sex.

In the responses printed here, you'll often notice that there is no indication of the writer's sex or that of the partner in question. Sometimes I can deduce the sex by the writer's Sexuality Forum previous postings. Often I can't. I have presented all comments here without my guesses, so you can play too. I think it's fascinatingly educational to read, for instance, a wonderful treatise of how to do oral sex on a man and not know if it is written by the man himself or by his partner, female or male.

It's also fascinating to read an array of sometimes contradictory hints and tips displayed here and realize that everything shared is the result of an individual's (often two individuals') personal experience. Sometimes several people have discovered the same thing and we might be able to generalize. For instance, responses from a wide variety of people indicate that anal sex is greatly facilitated by lots of communication and lots of lubrication. On the other hand, a very particular and personal predilection might work for you or a specific partner or it might not.

Even if a bit of shared wisdom is of no immediate use, isn't it interesting to hear secrets from the most private aspect of other people's lives?

There may be times after reading a contribution in these pages that you'll want to respond personally, add your own comments, or disagree, or propose another angle from which to see the topic under discussion. May I suggest that you open—or continue—the conversation with someone in your own real life: "I read a comment today that got me thinking. How do you feel about...?" We can all benefit by more honest discussion of sexual matters in the world. So, as you open the pages of this book, I entreat you not only to enjoy yourself, but to enjoy someone else as well.

CHAPTER 1

The Single State

Though prepackaged dinners for two and honeymoon vacation-special deals may rub in the notion that you are out of step with the rest of humanity if you are not paired like socks with another human being, don't be disheartened. Coupledom is simply not as universal as it sometimes appears to be. Although some are stuck alone unhappily, even temporarily, and know no way out of it, for others not being part of a couple is a chosen way of life, with many benefits of its own. For some, being single can be a state of preparation for a coupled commitment. For others, it's a time of renewal and recovery from one relationship, perhaps in anticipation of the next. This "between time" can be one of happy personal growth and discovery. Yes, it can be lonely with no Someone Special to hug, but that does not mean one must go hugless. Yes, being without a lover can be sexually frustrating, but being single does not mean life needs to be without pleasure.

On Being Single

For the newly single, the world can be a bewildering place. For the unwillingly single, it can be a sad and dreary state. For many others, living as an unattached individual is simply life—good, bad, and so-so. The following people comment on the single state for themselves and, possibly, for you.

The only time you feel alone is when your mind isn't occupied. Take it from someone eternally single. When you are occupying your mind with something interesting, you are too busy enjoying what you are doing to think, "Gee, this would be better if I had a partner." You might want to get out of the house and do activities that can be done alone—sculling, horseback riding, jogging, whatever. The point is, you will see other people doing the same thing alone, and won't feel like you are sticking out from the others. Sit at home watching the TV and movies, you'll see a lot of couples . . . and feel like you are the only single. It's not easy avoiding the "reminders" but if you can, keep your mind involved. . . . Remembering that there is more to life than a relationship can take some of the sting out of it.

———

Welcome to your new life! It can be anything you want it to be, only don't expect it to be anything if you wait for it to happen "to" you! Life will require that you search, experiment, learn, find disappointment and failure, get up and do it again. How many times have you said to yourself, "If I had it to do over again, I would do it this way?" Do it that way. If that doesn't work, look for another angle. Just don't wait for life to happen. Make it happen!

———

You start by living again. Get out of the house and get yourself involved in activities that will feed and nurture your spirit. Always wanted to learn how to ballroom dance? Now is the time. Think you've got a marathon in you? Start training. Interested in Thai cooking? Take a class. As you begin to nurture your own inner spirit, you'll begin to find satisfaction, pleasure, and purpose in life once more, and this will bubble forth from the well of your soul to those around you. Your happiness will be evident in the smile on your lips, the glow of your cheek, the sparkle in your eyes. Life will fill you with pleasure and your cup will runneth over. The most attractive people are those who are content within themselves and have something to give. Not those who seek to fill an emptiness within themselves with the shallow attention of others.

Be yourself, and don't settle for second best. Be prepared for highs and lows, to meet wonderful people and jerks. Be comfortable with staying in on the weekend and renting a movie. Be open and willing to meet different types of people.

Being alone exacerbated this very profound sense of being a pariah that I had while in high school. In retrospect, the pain was a great catalyst for change. When I'd absolutely had my fill, I was much more willing to assume risks, and do new things quite out of character to expand my horizons. Answering a personals ad was quite a radical departure from my usual take on social situations . . . but it is how my husband and I met.

If you crave touching, may I suggest a caring, nurturing massage? I experience the same need and, if chosen with care, a masseur can provide a satisfying and nonthreatening experience.

If you can find a "body pillow" (an oversized or tubular pillow) to "cuddle" with, you might not get that "all alone in bed" feeling. I don't have a big bed, just to avoid that feeling. Also, I suggest keeping the bed warm—don't skimp on sheets, comforters, or blankets. Nothing says "alone" like a cold bed and cold sheets. While we are talking, use comfortable sheets. Many times, I sleep in the buff on cotton sheets.

Not the same as the warm skin of a lover, but there is some comfortable sensation there. Better than nothing, eh?

———

Being lonely is something I have to deal with every day. I have engrossed myself in my work, for one. I even took a meaningless second job that keeps me out of the house for two nights during the week to cut down on the amount of time I spend alone. I guess a positive thing that has come from this is that I have learned other ways to occupy myself. I have some hobbies. I have also developed stronger ties with my family that in the past were lacking. I don't think there is any surefire way to stop from feeling lonely; it's human nature to feel that way. You just have to learn to be comfortable with your independence and try to concentrate more on any hobbies you may have or have always wanted to try.

———

You must take time off before jumping into another relationship. Find yourself, be with friends, and get out to help you heal faster.

———

The thing is to get a life with your own self first. If you don't have a life alone, what life would you have to share? Looking for the right partner to give you a life is a bit like putting the cart before the horse.

———

I have been single for the past year and a half and am having more fun than in my whole entire life. I used to sit around worrying about why I don't have a boyfriend, but now I am going out all the time and doing things I want and not worrying about someone else's schedule.

———

As a single guy, the commercial hype of Valentine's Day can make even the most well-adjusted and optimistic single person feel like a pariah. But it is important to ignore the hype, and I couldn't agree more with you on your suggestion to take stock of the important people who like you day in and day out. They are far more important and fulfilling than a fleeting mismatched romance. Having been in the two-by-two parade to board Noah's Ark with some pretty incompatible people in the past, I think I'll sit this one out.

I'm a fifty-four-year-old woman who recently withstood twelve years of celibacy. These were long years, encompassing what some say could be my most sexually powerful years. I am overjoyed to report that after moving to a large city on the east coast I have reawakened my sexual being. What I believe to be most true is that people (men, women, children) are attracted to vibrations, not to the physical trappings that the media tend to emphasize. It is the spirit that draws men to women, at least men worth knowing. Certainly sexual attracting and "dating" changes after a certain time. Yet I am now in a dynamite sexual and loving relationship with the most beautiful twenty-seven-year-old man, and I have no lack of male suitors whenever I decide to go out on the town. I believe in my beauty, my power, my attractiveness. I respect myself and demand that everyone I meet does as well. It is the human heart that is attractive, not weight or fashion or age. The only limitation is not imagining a dream that is big enough to encompass all that you wish for in life. P.S. Moving is certainly a key in this equation. Very often we stick with the familiar and become stuck. If you are not getting what you want, pick up and go to a place where the opportunities widen.

I am very proud to be single, especially when I think of many of my friends who are unhappy in relationships but not willing to take the risk of getting out of them. I am proud that I can be on my own and not succumb to the pressures of finding a mate. I admire those qualities in other people. Sometimes I look around and watch the couples playing their games and talking their talk. I don't want to play anymore. I'd rather not be dating than to go through the motions with some random fellow.

I can't for the life of me remember where I read this, but it's helped me immensely when those "I'll be alone forever" thoughts start crowding out everything else. Imagine that you are destined to fall in love with the absolutely perfect person for you, and that love will be reciprocated full force. There is no question that it will happen; the catch is that it will be another fifteen years (or ten or five, but in profound moments of panic, fifteen seems like the most appropriate number for this). So live the life you would live if you knew in your bones that this statement was true. You may meet a great partner much sooner, but in any case, you won't be lacking for a life well lived. I think the reason this works for me, psychologically, is that it removes the focus from being abandoned by the world to becoming an active planner and doer of life.

I'm still lonely at thirty, but I have certainly learned that I would much rather be lonely by myself than unhappy and lonely with the wrong person. I am on the heavy side, but I am discovering that it doesn't really make that much difference in meeting the type of quality people I want to associate with. I don't want to waste my time with someone who is highly concerned with superficial looks—I'm worth more than that. I actually find that I discriminate in the opposite way. If he or she is really physically attractive, I am much less apt to approach him or her without ever giving this person the opportunity to reveal his or her true self. Don't like to admit it, but it's true.

Sometimes I find one of the reasons I would like to have a girlfriend is that it would look better in front of others not to be single. Not that I am embarrassed being single, but to be single for a long time makes people think you really are unattractive, I think.

I can tell you, from experience, as soon as you make a goal for yourself, everything falls into two categories: success or failure. My opinion is to not "enter the market," so to speak. Just do your own thing, and let things happen as they come along. I know . . . sounds like Pollyannic BS. But, if you really feel like you haven't had much "experience" in attracting and snaring, why not get some? Find out what you like and enjoy, so you can find people with similar interests. Then do what you like and enjoy. Make friendships, because a good or great relationship (in my opinion) is a friendship taken to a deeper physically intimate level. Sure, there may be "fits and starts," but what in life doesn't have that? Making goals for yourself just puts on pressure to perform. Best thing you can do is relax as much as you can, and see what is out there for you. After that, you can decide there is nothing and alter your search, or you can decide there is something out there for you and pursue it. Remember the cardinal rule of the "single hunter": If what you are doing doesn't get you what you want, stop doing it and try something else.

The Sweetie Search

I get an inordinate number of letters and postings of the "Where can I find a great guy?" or ". . . meet other gay women?" or ". . . find someone to date?" variety. Alas, there is no orchard of ripening sweethearts in which you might wait with open arms for one to drop off the tree. Some people are lucky enough to fall for the girl or boy next door, the person in the next pew at worship service, the host's cousin at a friend's party. The rest of us who would like to have a sweetie need to get out and about and stay alert for possibilities . . . in other words, make our own luck. Yes, some people do seem born charmers, just as there appear to be natural athletes. Still, a person can learn how to be friendly (or at least appear to be), make casual conversation, move a budding friendship along to the desired state, and negotiate a relationship. Long years of professional experience have taught

me that for some, all of these interactions are bewildering and fraught with danger, while for others, they present an exciting challenge—like bridges to bungee
jumpers. Remember, for most people, attaining ease with
others is a process, not an innate gift. Start with something familiar and comfortable—an invitation to a
coworker to share lunch—rather than approaching an
attractive stranger in public, which appears to be some
sort of benchmark for the shy. That's a postgraduate level
exercise to which most of us don't even aspire! If you are
on a Sweetie Search, the least you can do is enjoy the
process.

I was struck by your phrase "Shyness is no more than exaggerated
self-centeredness." I've been working hard for the last seven years to
focus attention outward instead of inward. Now when someone asks
me, "How are you?" I say, "Fine. What's been happening with you?"
This turning the question or comment back to the person has not only
conquered a lifetime of shyness, but has made me realize that everyone
is looking for a listener, and that the good listener who really wants to
learn from others is always in demand. How I wish someone had
steered me to that realization sooner! It takes a lot of concentration
and practice, and I can still be stopped in my tracks by a direct question. The trick is moving continually to the other person instead of
focusing on your own thoughts and experiences. This needs as much
concentration as anything I've ever done in my life, but the rewards
are so bountiful that it is worth the effort.

———

It took five years since my last girlfriend to find this one. That's
over 1,500 straight nights of sleeping alone. The moral of my story: If
you are still searching, keep at it. You never know when or how luck
will find you. With me, it wasn't really "luck," because I had laid the

groundwork. It was more like fortune. It took my initiative (asking the first woman to dance) plus a little genuine luck (meeting my girlfriend through that woman just by chance). Finally the odds caught up with me.

———

I am a straight single male of forty-two, steady job, no criminal record, been told I'm cute. I, too, have asked women for that proverbial cup of coffee and seen quivering, stammering, stuttering recoils from supposedly intelligent, educated, baby-boomer women. When a man asks you out and you are not interested, a legitimate-sounding lie works best: "Thank you, but I'm already seeing someone." The man goes home with his dignity and gonads intact, not wondering what he supposedly did to scare the daylights out of you.

———

To those men who labor under the belief that women of a certain age (usually forty-plus) are no longer candidates for their attention, to all you guys who try to make conversation with me in coffee shops, who stare at me in stores, who say hi to me on the street, who compliment me on my clothes or my eyes or my smile, I've got news for you. I'm forty-eight years old.

———

Regarding the lady who's smart, attractive, interesting, 6 feet tall and still very single: I'm smart, ordinary looking, interesting, in my late thirties, 6-foot-4, and I've been dating shorter women of late because that's who's out there, not because I like the contrast. I would be absolutely delighted to meet a lady I could see eye to eye with, physically and figuratively, so put on your four-inch heels and when we see eye to eye introduce yourself. I've been to tall clubs too and been equally disappointed. It takes more than common altitude for two people to hit it off.

———

I am an attractive single gay woman who has long blonde hair and who wears skirts, high heels, and makeup to my professional job every day. I would like gay women to learn two important things: (1) You're never going to find me if you prejudge me. In other words, you're going to miss out on a lot of good lovers if you're only looking at women who look like stereotypical lesbians. (2) If you really want to stop others from discriminating against you, you should start by not discriminating against others. Even if I were heterosexual, you still shouldn't be thinking, "Straight little bitch!"

———

Yes, it seems most women prefer tall men. Except I wasn't looking for "most women," so I got involved in activities I enjoyed. I found one woman who not only prefers short men but is cute, sensitive, warm, fun to be with, helps me trigger earthquakes in our bed, and makes a nice income. We got married and she twisted her genes around mine to make one heckuva cute, funny, (and short) kid who's into sports and cooking.

———

This is an open letter to all the straight women in the city who have ever complained about the lack of decent guys. Women don't seem to grasp the concept of "Hey, make eye contact and smile." At minimum the world would be a brighter place if we all just realize that a smile does not mean any commitment whatsoever. If some guy takes your smile and wants to run the hundred-yard dash with it, and if he isn't the running partner you're looking for, just let him run on alone.

———

I wish I would meet women who don't feel put upon by guys asking them out, like they're doing you a favor by going out with you. And I also wish there were more women who are intelligent enough to realize that just because a guy asks them out, it does not mean that he wants to sleep with them that night. Guys can be simply friendly. And I wish there were more women who would do the asking out in the first place.

———

You can start by saying hi and then running out of the bar in embarrassment. Then work on not running out of the bar. Then work on saying, "Hi my name is..." It's not as bad as it sounds. Every journey begins with the first step and all that. It's just baseless fears that have to be overcome.

After fuming about being involuntarily sexless for a year or two I gave some serious thought to a blurb I read about men being interested in women who are interested in them. I tried approaching men as they do us (minus the sad attempts at witty lines) and, while I was occasionally turned away rather rudely (as some of us to do them), more often than not the reaction was favorable. This society is wrong in raising women to be passive and to be devastated by rejection. The platitude "Nothing ventured, nothing gained" is absolutely true.

I try to make sure that I have routine things that I do that force me to go out and socialize. Group sports that have a weekly schedule are good, as are courses. I have a set date with friends to meet Fridays after work for a drink.

I used to be scared, but no more, after I realized that we all want the same thing. A woman wants just as much love and attention and sex as us single guys do. It's their job to appear available, and it's our job to take them up on that by starting a conversation, no matter how uncertain we feel. When you feel like hanging back, ya gotta remember your role in the mating dance, and then go for it. Get over the hump.

At clubs when I talk to girls I compliment them on their hair or their nails and ask them where'd they get them done, like I want to be referred.

Frankly, there's nothing you can do but get with the program if you think someone is interested in you. Just say, "Hi, my name is. . ." If your perception was the least bit accurate, she'll at least give you her name back. If your perception wasn't accurate, you might try working on your perception skills.

———

Make it a point to say a friendly hello to at least six completely new women every day for a month. Not just to women you find cute, but any breathing woman, especially women you don't find attractive. Be sincere and friendly, and you will find you'll get a whole range of reactions. Since you weren't looking to flirt (which is why it helps to start with women you don't find attractive), you'll learn not to take personally the rejection or fearful or dirty looks from some, and you'll find some to be very friendly. It's like customer service—some people are just in a bad mood that day, and it doesn't have a thing to do with you.

———

I met my former husband at fifteen, married at nineteen, so I never dated. Didn't know how to meet or talk to men. So I joined a matchmaking service on the Net that was free. I got real used to getting rejected, learned how to make small talk, learned how to call men up on the phone because I didn't want to give them my number. It either works or it doesn't. I have made some really good friends this way, been terribly hurt (took it all too personally), and still can get to feeling that way. The feelings don't last as long nor do I take it so hard. That comes with experience. The Internet gave me a way to meet lots of guys who are also looking to meet someone to date. That's just how I did it. It's not easy for anyone.

———

Vulnerability is the name of the game . . . or maybe I should say openness. Sure it's awkward and you don't know what to say—but neither does she. Depending on the woman you're approaching, she may have been brought up to not make the first move—"It's not lady-like . . ."—or she may be feeling things out, be interested, but not have the nerve to say hello. I've decided sometime within the last thirty years that life is too short to not take chances. If I see a person who interests me, I will make it a point to say hello. That doesn't mean I'm going to throw myself all over this person, or ask him or her to come home with me for the night, but a simple hello isn't too risky.

I met my partner online about two years ago; we became very close friends at first and then slowly over time it became more than just a friendship. We began talking on the phone and after a year and a half of a long-distance relationship we made the decision that I would move halfway around the world to be together, and it was the best decision we could have made. We've been living together for almost six months now and know we want to grow old together. Just a word for those thinking about bringing an Internet relationship to reality: Make sure you really know each other more than just a few months; take advantage of the ability to "talk" over the Net. I know the communication we shared before taking this to the next level is what has made our relationship as strong as it is today.

I had a relationship with a man I met on the Internet. A few of my friends are very suspect of the entire process. They question why anyone would resort to this avenue. Personally, I find it much easier online to "weed out" the people who are less than good matches. If I spend several weeks or months e-mailing or chatting I can learn a great deal about a person. If his interests lean toward NASCAR, camping, and tobacco spittin' contests, we probably don't have much in common.

I went 3,000 miles to meet the other man in my life, and I am not sorry for one instant. You take a risk, with potential great rewards. Have you corresponded a lot with this person? I suggest going that route to better feel out the emotional terrain, before jumping on a plane or into the driver's seat. Maybe you will decide it's not worth the energy spent; maybe it will only make a stronger—and mutual—bond between you. Time and equal effort by both of you will help the right choice become evident.

———

If you're gong to run a personal ad, be willing to take a risk and make it real. "SWM seeks SWF; makes a great Veal Parmesan, will tolerate most chick flicks, promises never to run down her family if she'll promise to be nice to my brother at the annual family picnic. Happens to think that candlelight dinners and walks on the beach are overblown bits of Hallmark sentimental shtick, but admits that he's done both on occasion and enjoyed himself. Would settle for a glass of merlot and a good conversation." See . . . you get a feeling for the person. And meeting through the Net offers a great many advantages. It's relatively risk-free and you can spend some time getting to know the person before you ever have to come face to face for a drink or a meal.

———

Listen, and if someone brings up something that you are knowledgeable about or even just interested in, engage them in conversation. I have never met a person who does not want to talk about their own habits and hobbies.

———

The best way a girl can break the ice is to say, "Hi—mind if I sit down?"

———

If she keeps hanging around when there isn't anything to talk about she may be waiting for you to ask her out. If she seems to touch you, or invade your private sphere more than others would, she might prefer to be even closer to you. If she seems to give you more attention than others in the room she may think you are worth the attention . . . or she may just be being friendly. Don't know until you ask, unfortunately.

———

I think the best way to break out of a shell is to start talking to women. Start off with women you have no interest in whatsoever, just on a friendly basis. This will (1) get you practice in talking to women and (2) demonstrate to other women (whom you may be interested in) that you are a well-socialized, non-creepy guy. So relax, be yourself, and start with "Hi."

I hope someone sees me, thinks of me with speculative lust, and— gosh darn it- –will be brave and confident enough to come over and say hi.

I admire a man with the balls to come up to me and introduce himself. I will always talk to him, for at least a few minutes.

Where to Go A-Sweetie-Hunting

Given that there is no orchard of blooming Sweetie trees, here are some methods that have worked for others.

I would say decent-sized private parties are the best place to prowl for willing women. You have something in common by being there, the liquor is usually flowing, there are places to retreat to that might not be accessible at a club, and people in general seem friendlier at these types of social occasions than at a commercial establishment.

If you're a woman dying to meet a woman to have a relationship with, get yourself involved in a gay community, activity, or gay support group where you will be with people you won't feel uncomfortable about approaching to date.

Work is for work, and not for man-hunting. Why create waves where you work? If you and that person grow to have personal problems, you will still have to work with them every day. If you can handle that, then go ahead, but it is harder than you think.

———

I got severely burned by dating someone from work once. I still have to look at him every day, and he is a complete jerk. I would most definitely have forgotten him if I didn't have to deal with him at work. I will never fish off the company pier again, and would never, under any circumstances, recommend it.

———

In the past three months I moved to a new city, am active, but that lonely desperate feeling is tough to hide. I have had success keeping busy (basketball, beach volleyball, softball leagues), and my next step will be church.

———

Last January I joined a temple seeking spiritual guidance and, boy, I am surrounded by men of all ages. Even though I am not currently seeking a sexual partner, just being around all that testosterone makes me feel great.

———

Rather than the bar scene, do you belong to any organizations (non-business) where you have an opportunity to socialize? My friends keep telling me I need to find something I enjoy doing and do it; then I may meet someone with whom I share a common interest. Great, but how many men are into quilting and cross-stitch?

———

Since I'm a twenty-six-year-old guy in a college town, I go out, kind of hoping I might meet someone, and end up surrounded by nineteen-year-olds. To avoid that, I usually go to the bars and cafés on the townie end of town, farther from the campus. The bars aren't quite part of "the bar scene," but more mellow places where people go with their friends. I read and write in cafés, see bands at the rock and folk clubs in town, go to a reading every now and then. Eventually I start to see some of the same people around, which makes it a little easier to start up a conversation. Every now and then I go out on a date with someone I meet that way.

———

Are you getting out among a lot of people? What I mean is, Do you have a job? Go out with friends? Volunteer your time in a hospital or civic organization where you come into contact with a lot of different people? (Believe it or not, I met my late mate doing volunteer work.) Besides, just being married doesn't guarantee instant happiness.

———

Join clubs, get a part-time job, talk to the people in your dorm. Things "clique up" surprisingly fast on a college campus, so the best advice I could give you is never to limit yourself to the immediate circle of friends you will soon find yourself in. They will, of course, be fine people, but never again will it be as easy to meet so many new people as in the first few weeks of college. Seize every single opportunity you can; think in terms of making friends rather than landing a boyfriend (this includes making female friends as well). Try not to prejudge people; ask questions and listen to the answers. Take one class every semester that is totally different from the rest of your schedule. I found that those invariably ended up being not only the most interesting (because everything is new and unfamiliar), but contained the most people whom I didn't know, and hence lots more opportunities to meet new people.

———

Try new things all the time. If you can't make up your mind about something, pick the opportunity that is most foreign or different, provided the new choice is reasonably sane, of course. You will learn a lot and have a blast. If you make a new friend or a boyfriend, that's a bonus, but in any case, you'll learn something new and hence won't feel like you "failed" because you didn't meet the all important goal of

Bringing a Boyfriend Home from College to Tell All Your Friends About. Hell, don't even view that as a goal, if you can help yourself.

———

It's just a numbers game. And you can't win if you don't play.

———

Miraculous things happen if you keep yourself open to them.

CHAPTER 2

The Dating Game

Although some people call Sweetie Hunting a game, there are no rules, and, unlike in anything played with lots of running feet and a ball, it's possible for everyone involved to win. A date is an exploration, each meeting determining if both parties would like to know more. Who calls, who pays, who makes the first social or sexual move are all up for grabs and open to discussion. Part of the information exchange that needs to take place in the earliest interactions reveals what you require from a friend/lover, and that information exchange can be as much of a learning experience about yourself as it is for and about a potential partner. In essence, it's a verbal manual on The Care and Feeding of Me. If she describes herself as "old-fashioned," don't wait for her to phone you for a date. If he says he's "not available for a relationship right now," believe him and move on or prepare to be a buddy. When no indication of what is wanted is provided, rather than trying to figure out the "right" way, please yourself. Since dating is called a game, play at it. Don't make it into work.

The Shopping Process

If an intimate relationship is what you want, what a pity that you can't just jump into the middle of one with an agreeable partner. In order to find someone special in your life, if that's what you're looking for, some winnowing must take place—in person, online, via matchmaking services or friends, or all of the above. Like with car buying for those who hate to shop, some preparation and effort just can't be avoided. So go ahead, kick the tires, but while you're at it, as I've said before, remember to enjoy yourself . . . and enjoy someone else too.

Dating does not always lead to sex! Dating is a way to make new friends and enjoy people in a social setting. Start there. Tell one or two people you know that you want to date. They may be able to introduce you to someone. If they do, *go!*

———

Once I've exchanged numbers with someone I prefer to call or be called within twenty-four hours of the exchange. That way the circumstances/the moment is fresh in my mind and hopefully in his or hers. I find that in waiting the moment, feelings, and context are lost, and the first few minutes of the phone call are an awkward catch-up game: "Hi, I'm Suzy. Yes, Suzy Q, and we met Thursday of last week at Lala's party and I was wearing blah, blah and you said blah. . . ."

———

Go for broke. Invite her to dinner at a nice restaurant and have a nice, long chat. She will get the idea that you are interested, and she will make it clear, one way or another, whether she is interested in pursuing the matter. If she is, great. If not, you've had a nice dinner and a nice conversation!

———

For a single guy having a tough time getting a date, and finding that every female seems to have a boyfriend, it's easy to fall into misogyny and the stereotypes that accompany it. Guys start to think how easy it is for a woman to get laid, how if only a woman were as interested in having sex and intimacy as we were, we men wouldn't need to play games in order to get what we want. Then we could both cut to the chase and build a relationship. If we lonely men can't get a date it must be the women's fault; the women only want jerks. They only want shallow rich guys. They want sex, but won't admit to it, and on and on. This is an endless loop. If we can't get a date, we get a little anti-female, which makes the guy a little less attractive, making it harder to get a date, which makes us more willing to believe women are against us, making us more anti-female, making us more unattractive, which . . . well, you get the idea.

———

Guys (in general, not all) aren't good at reading implied feelings; we need to be told what you want and how *you* interpret things. An agreement shared by and followed by two people is a code of ethics. An assumption made by one and not discussed with the other is blind faith.

———

We met in person after a year and four months of chatting online. I know that seems like a long time to most, but I suppose it was a comfort-level thing on my part. It took a long time of just talking and getting a realistic sense of each other online (and in some phone conversations) before I felt comfortable seeing her in person. When I finally did it was surreal. On the one hand, I had to get used to just *being* around her for the first time. I had to get used to her mannerisms, the way she talked, the way she observed the world around her. On the other hand, I was completely comfortable with her. There was no "blind date" awkwardness. We knew where each other's head was.

———

In my experience, it's a fine line to walk on a first date between not talking enough about yourself and talking too much about yourself.

I've heard complaints on both sides from women talking about their first dates. Focus on the strong points about yourself and stay away from the negative until you know each other better. If I were with a woman who wanted to unload a lot of her past or tell me more than I really wanted to know the first time out I'd think there was a chemistry problem, too. We all expect our date to put their best foot forward on a first date, and if she's saying something negative about herself, I'd wonder what was worse that she wasn't telling me already. It's good to be honest with someone, warts and all, but not right away. You have to ease them into it after they've seen some of the good things about you.

———

To tell you the truth, if I really like a girl and we're going out and we are both attracted to each other, I am just upfront and honest with them. "I want to be intimate with you" ... or, "I am really attracted to you and I want to be with you." You'd be surprised how often a little honesty can go along way. Most of the time they want the same things we do.

———

Look, I'm a shy guy and I'm slow, but if I'm really attracted to a girl and it's the third or fourth date, I'm ready to kiss her. If she avoids the kiss and doesn't explain why, then I interpret it to mean she's not really attracted to me, and I lose interest in her.

———

When I have a choice in partners, I'm much more relaxed about the dating game than when I have no choice. No reason to worry, right? It's like sex—when you are getting it, it isn't a big deal. When you aren't, it is! Or, maybe you are concerned that you don't want to waste this time of many opportunities. You want to get the "right one." I'd say, take a look at all of them, pick a first and a second choice, then start up a friendship and see what happens. If it leads to a relationship, go through with it. If it leads nowhere, try out choice number 2. Don't get focused on the future. Don't go out with anyone with the idea that it will, or should, "go somewhere." Just enjoy the time with this person, as you would a friend. That way, your head is clear. If you aren't planning ahead, you aren't . . . planning ahead. You relax. Things work their own way, and that is that.

———

Nothing says a first date has to end with a hot kiss. I saw a show one time where this guy was very successful with women. He never gave a full-blown kiss on the first date. He would take the woman's hands in his, look into her eyes and tell them how much he enjoyed her company, then give her a kiss on the cheek and that was it. The women loved it. Too often we expect too much from that first meeting. I know at one time I spent so much time during the date wondering how it was going to end that I didn't enjoy the date itself. If you go into it knowing how you are going to handle it (as in the example above) you can just relax about it. And just a hint, guys: We can tell when you think that you are owed something because of "good" behavior! Hoping you're going to get physical is fine (that's what I might be thinking too!), but expecting it or getting angry when you don't makes me feel like I'm just an object. The direct method is usually a turn-on for me if we've been getting along so far, or at least it allows me to decline or accept gracefully!

Turn-ons

The French say *"chacun a son goût,"* which translates roughly as "different strokes for different folks." Nowhere is this more noticeable than in sexual attraction. You take notice of that person over there, while someone else is interested in exploring what's possible with this one here. Following is a variety of responses to "What turns you on?"

To me it is a man with self-confidence, self-knowledge, and the ability to laugh. I love those little laugh lines around a man's eyes and to see them crinkle and his eyes light up when he sees me. A self-confident man gets me every time, especially if he isn't arrogant but sure.

———

A nice big ... brain. Creativity and intelligence, together with a healthy body.

———

I love to talk with my lover about anything and everything. So being intelligent and having a good sense of humor and good communication skills are all essential. Someone sensual and passionate, kind, compassionate, thoughtful ... unconditional love and acceptance, great kisses and soft touches and strokes.

———

What's sexy to me is nice broad shoulders tapering to a narrow waist with a tight set of buns, well-developed deltoids, really well-shaped lips, a man's hands, eyes that have that soft seductive look.

———

I love a man's hands and forearms, shoulders, back. One of the most steamy things I remember from a movie is when a man held a woman by gently resting his hands on her bare back as they were dancing.

———

What's a turn-on is the whole person, the aura they present, the sexuality that seeps from every inch of their body.

———

Sexy is someone who enjoys who they are and what they look like. They try to show off their good traits to me and enjoy looking at mine. I think my boyfriend is incredibly sexy because although he may be starting to get a little belly, he has this awesome hard chest and loves to flaunt it.

———

To me sexy is a man who knows how to treat a lady, holds the door for her, calls her "Darling," brings her flowers every once in a while, and the *sexiest* thing he can do is tip his Stetson to her and flash that sexy grin! That is melt city for me!

There's something about a girl in a baseball cap and ponytail that really does it for me.

The physical part is probably the least of it to me. Intelligence is very sexy to me, so is a sense of humor (one with a little attitude is nice). Self-assured without being stuck up is also sexy.

Now if you want to talk physical, there's *nothing* like a nice pair of legs in a short skirt.

Sexy for me is a way of thinking. I've seen unattractive men who are very sexy. The way they carry themselves, confidence, sensitivity. It's a mental thing 80 percent of the time.

The things that I find to be very sexy in men is a certain way of holding themselves, as if they like being in their own bodies. A man who can be sensual, especially with his own body, who likes touching himself, that is very sexy—better yet, touching another man in a sensual way. It's rare to see since even gay porn doesn't show much in the way of sensuality.

A few things: Self-confidence. . . . A great ass (for boys). . . . A beautiful smile. . . . A lovely overall shape (for girls). . . .

I'm a sucker for a great smelling man; men's fragrances just seem to intoxicate me. A well-trimmed beard, but specifically a goatee. I'm a sucker for facial hair. An attractive mouth—full lips and white teeth. Hygiene is a *major* turn-on for me.

———

Watching a man use his hands. It's not that important what his hands may be doing—working on something, playing around unconsciously with his keys, rubbing his arm, buckling his belt, slicing, dicing, and kneading dough in the kitchen (*love* that!), massaging something. Those hands just mesmerize me, and the tension builds delectably!

———

Eye contact that is part of a clever, demure look that says, "I know what you're thinking and I'm thinking it too."

———

If a woman gives me her full attention it makes me feel like I am the most important person to her. Insecurities are gone and I am hers.

———

Little things do it. The hair things. All of it. The wiggle. The slow blink with those gorgeous eyes. The drinking from a straw thing. Finger on the rim of a glass. A friendly, loving touch.

———

Long hair ... a seductive look ... a teasing kiss where she pulls back as our lips *just* begin to touch ... another seductive look ... to hear her say, "I want you to fuck me" ... to feel her rub my nipples through my shirt ... oh god, after that I'm gone!

———

A smile from a sexy girl.... A cute belly button poking out a half shirt.... Dancing.

———

Coffee on lazy Sunday mornings.... Abstinence for longer than a day or two at a time.

———

Turn-offs

"They don't seem to notice I'm alive," and "I never seem to get a second date!" are common plaints. Here is an assortment of traits and characteristics that put some people off. Look in the mirror, review your last dismal flirt attempt, and, if you're one of the bewildered also-rans, perhaps something here will suggest why.

Driving in a very unsafe manner; being rude to service staff; an obvious lack of respect for significant women in his life such as mother or sisters.

Refusal to talk for days on end and refusal to explain why.

The smell of excessive alcohol, not taking the time to make sure both of us give and receive some pleasure, a guy without a backbone.

Lack of cleanliness, smoking, poor manners, too much make-up, snobbishness or elitism, bigotry, lack of a certain level of intelligence.

Men who reek of cheap cologne and use lame lines to hit on women. Men whose eyes undress every other woman in the vicinity as he's talking to me. Men who talk to my breasts (although if I'm married to that man this is perfectly acceptable, especially if he says, "And are you two happy today?"). And yes, of course, men who run down their last partner.

A woman who expects me to pay the bill just because I'm a man. I'm happy to pay; I am a gentleman after all, but it feels a bit strange in these days to date someone who never even tries to reach for her money.

I find that *whining* is a huge turn-off. There is nothing more unattractive than a woman who spends her time complaining about her life, her surroundings, men. This is a clear sign of an unstable person. Tragic storytelling is also a turn-off, for example, the worst date I ever went on was with a girl who spent forty minutes telling me about her ex-boyfriend and what an jerk he was, how he cheated on her, how he stole her car, blah blah blah. People have to realize if you want to make a good impression, you must keep a positive outlook on life, no matter how hard it is. Life is only as hard as you make it for yourself.

———

A big turn-off is women who can't put themselves together. I don't mean put on a $500 Prada skirt and seven layers of make-up. Just try to be feminine. Wear what looks good on you, try to accentuate your best features. I can't stand women who walk around like they just woke up and grabbed whatever dirty laundry was on the floor and walked out the door.

———

Smoking, excessive drinking, wearing old clothes that are out of style, hairstyle that's out of style, and dancing like a fool are things that immediately turn me off. I won't even give him a chance.

———

I am turned off by women who don't have a good sense of humor. That's extremely important to me. Smoking is a turn-off, but if a woman doesn't smoke around me I am fine with it. A woman who never offers to help pay a bill when we go out I think is very selfish. (Of course, I would always say no thank you if they did, but it's considerate to ask.)

———

I am a man and I am not going to have any kind of romantic relationship (with or without sex) with any woman if that woman still has romantic relationships with other people. I am not going to date anyone who even has a slight romantic feeling toward others. I always keep a distance with my female friend because it makes me feel very uncomfortable to get too close to a woman and yet not have a romantic relationship with her. My standard has nothing to do with morality; this is about dignity. I feel that my dignity will be torn apart if I have a close relationship with a woman who also has romantic feelings toward others.

Friends and Lovers

If your old pal suddenly seems strangely desirable, do you want to risk fooling with the friendship? The continuum of relationship types is often as fluid as that of sexual orientation. Just as there is a huge amount of variation between the two poles of heterosexuality and homosexuality, there may be an even larger array of possibilities between friend and lover. Don't give up a promising interaction because it doesn't fall neatly into conventional boxes. Create your own.

I have many women friends, just a few of whom have become lovers. I have never had sex with a woman who was not a friend first, and except in a very few cases has remained a friend after the sexual relationship had come to an end. I recommend this approach; it is very satisfying and elevates the importance of friendship.

———

Sex can be destructive to a relationship if the two people involved aren't on the same wavelength as to what the sex means. If one is seeing it as something that's moving the relationship forward into something deeper, and the other person is just assuming that it's a "just for fun" type situation, it can completely destroy the friendship. I actually discussed this the other day with one of my guy friends. We talked about why, when the chemistry is there between us, we didn't have sex when given the opportunity. Both of us came to the conclusion that we couldn't do it because in some ways we felt that it would actually devalue our friendship, and if one of us decided we wanted more than the other, we'd have an awkwardness in our relationship that would be destructive.

If you have friends whom you can have sex with, wonderful! But you both have to understand that's exactly what it is, just sex, not a mutually exclusive relationship. (Unless of course, you both decide that's the direction you want the relationship to take.)

I started a job working in an office of several women, one of whom I couldn't stand in the beginning. Not attractive, always making cutting remarks, that kind of thing. After about a month I found myself wanting to be working in the same workspace as this woman as often as possible. I found her cutting remarks to be more like my sometimes-sarcastic sense of humor; we could tease each other mercilessly and never be offended by it because we knew the context it was coming from. This in turn, for some reason, made her more physically attractive to me. We ended up being very close friends, going to a park after work and just having a beer and talking. I was going through a divorce at the time, but she was married, so it never went past that . . . although I wish it would have. It does, however, address the question of whether a man can be attracted at all after initially not seeing *anything* in a woman to begin with.

My best friend and I have been friends for eleven years, and we have always had a platonic relationship. We have always had common friends among us, but we share a certain intimacy that we don't have with anyone else. We have always been there for each other, have fought and made up, traveled together, and seen each other through bad relationships. We have had flirtations but nothing further from that. All our friends say than we should just get married and get it over with, even her mom tells us she wants me to be her husband so she can stop dating all those losers. I do feel that if we took the whole relationship road it would derail our friendship, and that's a risk I'm not willing to take.

———

I have a female friend of four years or so with whom I definitely have a platonic intimacy. She can tell me things she can't tell her boyfriends. She usually falls asleep early in the evening, so when I come over, she'll change into her nightgown and we'll watch TV until I leave. At times, she has sort of flirted with me, nothing physical, more intimate. However I know she has zero interest in me "in that way," probably never will. But we fit so well and that's what a relationship is, right?

———

During my adult life, most of my very best friends have been women. Only a few of them have been lovers. But every one of the lovers was a friend first and, in most cases, a friend afterward. I wouldn't have it any other way.

Nice Guys

Over the years this topic has stirred up more irate mail than practically any other (except maybe human-animal sexual contact). All these "nice guys" (who come across, more often than not, as angry and whining in their letters, and not nice at all) cursing women for not appreciating their good qualities while those same women are crying on their kindly available shoulder about the guys who done them wrong—who are, of course, the ones they find attractive. Perhaps some insight lies in the exchanges below?

A lot of the women who tell men they are "too nice" actually mean that the men are too dull. There *is* a difference. For the record, I am attracted to guys who are a little bit shleppy and neurotic. The macho bad boys love themselves so much I feel they don't really need me.

———

When "Mr. Nice Guy" asked his women friends for a list of his attractive qualities they said, "Intelligent, funny, easy to talk to, and very sweet." Did anyone say "Good-looking, physically fit, well-dressed"? There are guys out there who do not have a clue that some of us care what they look like! Character is important, but it's not the first thing you notice about a prospective date. Studies have shown that for most couples both people are in the same range of physical attractiveness. That would suggest that the majority of women choose their men at least partially for their looks. Maybe your correspondent is not sufficiently self-aware to realize that he's going after women who are a lot better looking than he is.

———

Many of the men who complain that they can't get a date because "women only go for jerks" have it backward. What is really going on is that the men who are saying this are men who only go for women who like men who act like jerks. And guess what! Most of these women are jerks! For the most part, these men are going after women based mostly on looks, and those model types turn them down because (big surprise!) they are also going for men based on looks. So the men turn away rejected, not realizing that if they tried to find a woman based on her personality they might find someone who isn't looking for a jerk.

———

One more hit on the Nice Guy Syndrome. It's what I call the Betty and Veronica story. Veronica was beautiful, self-centered, and deceptive. She was also the desired one. Betty, although also pretty (after all, a guy drew the comic), was down-to-earth, self-reliant, and trustworthy, everybody's pal. As much as men say women want to get jerked around, I've watched some men complain about game playing then lap it up as some pretty, vapid phony pours it on. The stereotypes work both ways, fellas.

———

It's very difficult to know when a woman is interested in me. After an evening with women friends I often hear later from one that another had been flirting with me. I thought she was just friendly. Vague hints are just not real communication in these supposedly liberated but politically volatile times. We all know that women are tired of getting "hit on." I hear much complaining about the quality of men in conversations with women, and I generally agree with them, yet it seems that most women have never asked a man out on a date. I would think that if a woman were interested in finding non-typical males she would make a point of asking out a nice guy. Doesn't coyness and passivity increase the likelihood that she will end up with the very type of male she complained about? Have the Sexual Revolution and the Women's Movement had any impact on the search for romance between men and women? Why don't more women walk their talk and act liberated in regards to dating? We "sensitive guys" who have gotten the message aren't dating much because we are less likely to initiate. I am getting extremely lonely while being respectful of women's boundaries.

"I'll Call You"

Being told "I'll call you" and then never hearing another word is such a common complaint for those who are dating that I have several times run whole columns on this phenomenon, inviting men (usually, but not always) who have ever practiced this cowardly kiss-off to say why they did. If you're waiting for a phone call that never comes, you're unlikely ever to know the reason. Why not choose an explanation that comforts you (like "I was just too much woman for him!") rather than one that causes you pain?

Why do I say I'll call then don't? In the warmth of the moment I do want to, but later I realize I don't want to.

———

Although I have never said, "I'll call you" after sex and didn't, I have said it under other circumstances and failed to follow through. In general I did so (1) because I wanted to keep my options open and knew that I was bad at snap evaluations, (2) I figured that my counterpart was as capable of operating the telephone as I was, and (3) calling someone who I'm attracted to but don't know very well is uncomfortable and therefore easy to postpone ... indefinitely. I recognize that number 2 reveals some naiveté regarding our culture's social expectations, but I remain confused. I once said I'd call to a woman where there was, I thought, some mutual attraction, but events interceded and I began another relationship. I'm not entirely comfortable with not calling the first woman back, but calling someone to tell them you really like them but are actually dating someone else seems awkward. I'm not sure it would be appreciated.

———

Dating is not a lifetime commitment or even a temporary one. It is a conditional one that either party can put an end to without notice or explanation, even if sex is involved. The idea that men are rude because they don't call back is just silly. If the date were a wretched experience for the woman, she wouldn't want the man to call. Doesn't the man have the same option? If the woman wants another date, why doesn't she make the call? The man may have been left with the impression that she had a lousy time; he wants to avoid the pain of rejection. Even if she said she had a good time he may not have believed her; women often send conflicting messages. So if you're a woman cursing men while sitting by the phone on Friday night, stop obsessing about what might have been, and move on with your life.

———

So why doesn't a man call a woman after he says he will? He really *is* a total idiot and waited too long. He's married. He felt passion for the moment . . . only.

———

I think women are often reluctant to say to men, "Look, this isn't working out" because men often don't take that kind of rejection well. They get angry; they say mean things. So a woman learns (to everyone's detriment, I believe) to avoid that kind of directness. I think men are often reluctant to initiate what could be a difficult or messy emotional conversation because they're often not comfortable operating on that plane. They're willing to do it to make a relationship work, but what's the point if you've decided the relationship is over, or is never going to progress any further or deeper? So they take the easy way out, the coward's way out.

———

I think that sometimes people try on words for size the same way you might try on a coat or a pair of shoes. "Let me see how this fits, let me say how it looks and feels on me." A man starts seeing you, and he wants to be in love with someone in his life; he wants to have someone to make future plans with. He wants to be not just dating but to be in a serious relationship. Maybe he's been in one or two of those before in his life, so he knows how to act in one; he knows the things you're supposed to say. So he talks about future things you might do together and gives you compliments, and maybe even says he loves you . . . but maybe he's only seeing how those words sound, or trying to decide how much truth there is to them, or feeling you out to see how you'll respond or whether you're interested in the same things he's interested in. Or maybe he's only saying those things because he wants to have sex with you. Or, more likely, as soon as he achieves the goal of sex, he can see you more clearly (not because you haven't been there all along, but because his view of you has been fogged by his own romantic and sexual desires); and once he sees you clearly, he decides that he doesn't really want to pursue further interaction with you. But of course he's embarrassed because he's been leading you on to believe that he was thinking just the opposite. And rather than take responsibility for that change of heart or those misleading messages, he simply runs away.

———

The first (and only) time that we went out together she told me that she was living with her boyfriend. I assumed this was her way of letting me know that she wasn't interested so I didn't call again.

———

I don't call because I am embarrassed. I don't know what to say, or I fear that anything I might say would seem to be hurtful or insulting, and I don't know how to deal with the woman's anger or hurt. "I enjoyed our sex the other night but I am … married, engaged, going steady, gay, not interested in you." "The sex was fun but you are too fat, thin, short, tall, smart, dumb, old, young." "It wasn't fun. The sex was too fast, slow, messy, hard, too much work, boring." "I did it just to see if you would; I don't care for you." "I don't date sluts who have sex on the first date." How could I say any of these things to a woman? Yet it has to be one of these reasons. If he did like her and want to see her again, he would call.

———

I once dated a woman who asked me to promise to tell her when I felt the relationship was over and not just disappear. One night I fell asleep during dinner together at a restaurant. I told her that seemed a sign to me that the relationship was over. Can you guess what happened next? She blasted me, calling me egotistical and arrogant. I listened to a half-hour tirade very politely and we went home separately. I've told many friends this story and the universal response is, "What did you expect?" If you think she was an exception, think again. You'll never be able to give honest advice that says, "When a lover tells you why they are leaving, make sure you don't get angry at them for telling you; otherwise they will never tell anyone else in the future." The lesson I've learned is to say, "I'll call you" when it's a lie.

———

As to "I'll call you" I plead guilty, but for every failure on my part to carry through at least three rejections result when I do call women who, initially at least, exhibit great enthusiasm for me to do so. If I was not met over the phone with hostility, suggesting I was stupid to think she would lower herself to date me, I've gotten, at various times, the same excuses men gave you—went back to an old boyfriend, decided there was no likelihood of compatibility, didn't want involvement right now. It annoys and hurts us just as much as it does you women who have your own Big Lies and Cowards' Kiss-offs.

———

Why men don't call: One reason is "I lost your number." Why don't women presume moral innocence? Or if I say I'll call and I don't, why not call me? Another possibility is "I got really busy" or "A parent died but I still plan to call," "I'm shy," or "I didn't think you liked me." Women should and do have the right to make a phone call just as much as men do, so why do so few women bother? I am engaged and very happy because last year an ex-girlfriend *called me.* I had sent her a birthday card every year, but last year I forgot. She noticed.

Aha! Sex!

Eventually, sometime during the dating process sex is going to rear its head, preferably as a longed-for event, but sometimes as a dropped second shoe ("Uh oh, I was afraid this would come up!"). There are absolutely no rules here either about when, how, or who, no "best time to bring it up," no "third date dictum." There are friendships that include sex and those that don't. There are sexually exclusive arrangements and those more flexible. Sex for some is merely invigorating play, for others a demonstration of a deeply committed union. You can have whatever you and your partner agree upon. The only requisite is that you must talk about sex at some time. What does it mean to you if we do it? Will I lose your interest if I don't? What about disease protection? Rather than being an embarrassing ordeal that must be endured for the sake of the potential prize at the end, this verbal interchange can actually be an enjoyable part of the developing intimacy. For me personally, this sexual information dialogue is exactly how I define foreplay.

Moving toward physical affection, whether it's holding hands or rolling about on the floor, is not necessarily a sign of disrespect. Yes, you want to go slowly, but how else to test the waters of what's possible than seeing her reaction to you physically?

———

If I had a first date with a man and there were definite sparks, and he didn't make a move for sex, there would be no problem with me. I would take it as a sign that he is a decent guy who is interested in things other than getting laid, a guy with some class. I wouldn't think too much of it. Actually I would be quite put off if a man made a move to get sexual early on. Don't get me wrong; I'm not totally against physical stuff early on, but definitely no oral sex or intercourse in the beginning. If you want to wait for a while, more power to you. You'll probably have a better chance of getting busy with her later on too.

———

If I were attracted to a guy on a first date, felt tingly, and he didn't make a move, I might be a little disappointed. However, I would also feel that he respected me enough to wait. I see nothing wrong with getting in a lip lock on the first day if the chemistry is right. On the other hand, thinking about that first kiss, anticipating it can be very exciting.

———

You've got to think about the specific man you're with and the specific time of your life you're in (frisky, monogamous, serious) to figure out when to sleep with a guy. It's admittedly hard to hold out. But if you can look at waiting as part of the unbearable pleasure, maybe you can psyche yourself for a real treat after about four or five dates. On the other hand, some dates are just, clearly, about sex. Sure, there's always the twang of attachment, but if we're all being honest with ourselves, we know if a guy's a fling or the real thing. Think also about what you're looking for or in the mood for right now. The full feast— or just dessert?

———

A kiss helps a guy know a girl is interested in him. It encourages the guy to want to know and be with the girl. It's OK to say no to sex, but to avoid a kiss and a hug . . . well, a guy needs to feel the girl's skin and body and lips. It's one way for a guy and girl to find out if there is a potential relationship.

———

I don't think that a woman "owes" a man a goodnight kiss. I think that too many rules can spoil just about anything.

———

A squeeze and eye contact while holding hands, a sincere hug, a "Thanks, I had a nice time, would you like to . . . (insert: go to a movie next week, come over for dinner)?" You know, take a little initiative. Let him know that the lack of a kiss does not mean there's no interest.

———

With my ex, we were married before we had sex. In the case of my current S.O. she was interested in sex long before I was. She was ready on our second date (which was a campout, and her idea). I was not ready after five weeks of dating (but did anyway. Needed the outlet. Sort of wish I hadn't). So, each of us must decide on our own when we are ready. Don't try to use someone else's opinion to make yours.

———

I need to have an intellectual and emotional connection first to feel ready for the "Big Do." That also means that by this time I sense a spark. He has to have looked me dead on with "I want you" eyes. Of course, this could be two weeks, or two minutes, depends on the man.

———

My experiences with female and male have been basically the same. I don't read other people well when it comes to sexual attraction. I have always waited patiently, quietly and pleasantly going insane until the ton of bricks finally hit me that he or she might be interested in me too. I have always hated sexual wolves, so I have not often made the first move.

———

Just because you kiss doesn't mean you have to have sex. She needs to set limits she is comfortable with so she can decide ahead of time how physically intimate she wants to be. Then she can relax with the kissing and making out, draw the limits for the guy, and most guys would respect her limits. Have fun. Kiss the toads! No warty toad ever became a handsome prince without being kissed!

CHAPTER 3

Coupling

When I was growing up, the acknowledged life choices for women were "married with children" or "not yet so." One could always be "a career gal," of course, but it was never seen as a choice, simply what was available to a pitiable female whom no one asked to marry. Today life's possibilities have expanded for everyone. Any two people can form a couple. Their arrangement can include living together or not, with or without legal sanction, with or without children, with or without sexual exclusivity. No one will argue a frequent nostalgia for gentler times, but the twenty-first century does bring with it a much welcome romantic and sexual freedom of choice.

On Relationships

Some of the wisest words I know on making satisfying connections come from communications pioneer Virginia Satir. Although her focus was on enhancing self-esteem, I can't think of a better template for a happy relationship than Satir's Five Freedoms. Each person in the relationship must have "the freedom (1) to see and hear what is here, instead of what should be, was or will be, (2) the freedom to say what one feels and thinks instead of what one should, (3) the freedom to feel what one feels, instead of what one ought, (4) the freedom to ask for what one wants instead of always waiting for permission, and (5) the freedom to take risks in one's own behalf instead of choosing to be only 'secure' and not rocking the boat." (from *Making Contact*, Berkeley, CA: Celestial Arts, 1976.)

I don't think it's like riding a bike. Bikes are pretty much all the same; with few exceptions, if you can ride one you can ride them all. With relationships, practice helps—but every relationship presents new challenges. I would liken it more to learning a new piece of music if you're a musician. Some things you've learned from pieces you've played before will apply to the new one. Some won't. Some passages in the new piece will throw you completely, but only at first, and some will keep throwing you for years. Of course, when a piece of music throws you, you don't get hurt nearly as much as when a bike throws you. Maybe we should say starting a new relationship is like taming a new wild animal—experience helps, but you should expect to be surprised (pleasantly), puzzled, and possibly hurt.

———

If you can stand being alone, it's a good chance you are ready for a relationship, not desperate for one. That's the test. Make sure you're in a relationship because you want to be in one, not because you *need* to be in one. If you are doing things with your new guy you rarely do with other people, that's probably a good sign; it means you've found a relationship different from the others. Have you ever felt this level of nervousness that you'd screw it up? If not, that's another good sign. Your subconscious is probably recognizing a good thing when it sees it. The more you do in your relationship the more normal and natural it will become. You'll be able to speak your mind, and not worry how it will come out.

———

I think we as a society have a lot of romanticized ideals about marriage. One of them is the notion of lifelong marriages. Although I do feel many people are interested in and capable of lifelong marriage, I don't think its as easy as in the past. Most lifelong marriages weren't as long as they'd be today. Many men had more than one wife in their lifetimes because their first wife died during childbirth. Some women had more than one husband because a husband died prematurely. Before the Industrial Revolution, most people farmed the land and had to depend on the strong bond of marriage and shared tasks to remain fed and sheltered. Life revolved around the home and family, and opportunities to pursue outside activities were limited. Today we have many more opportunities to learn, travel, and do things totally unrelated to our daily lives. I think these days the *necessity* to remain married isn't there, and the opportunities to do otherwise are greater. I feel the reasons people used to stay married for a lifetime were due to a great degree on the circumstances of their lives as opposed to any great commitment.

———

I am in a new relationship of two months' duration. The leadership role gets assumed by the person who has the most at stake for a "thing" to get done. It all works out. Leadership is balanced I believe by both. Is the leader the one that says, Let's go in this direction, or the one who digs in the heels and refuses? In my case I find that we have to work at communication a lot! We differ greatly in our perceptions of the same thing, so I need to recognize that and ask him how he sees things. It amazes me how different we are, but I do see us as equals overall. We just have different needs. What really matters is knowing each other. Takes a heckuva lot of work, at least in my camp.

One day I came home and he was cleaning the oven. Upon questioning, he responded saying, "I was pissed because the oven was dirty and then decided if it was so important for me to have a clean oven and not so important to you, then maybe I should just do it myself." Now that kind of decision making and taking the lead is just fine with both of us. Buying cars and household items, paying bills, going on vacation, dealing with families, all the important stuff is shared via discussion first.

Unless you are committed to some unforeseeable obligation like taking care of an invalid or a baby, the amount of time you have to spend on anything including your relationship is the result of choices you have made and continue making.

You can have love without sex. You can have sex without love. You can have sex with one and love another. But to have sex and love together with one person is probably the best feeling in life.

How do you know you are in love? Looks to me like you get a clearer idea whether you are or not when the going gets rough. Then, if you want to change the other person or bail out of the relationship or kill yourself or otherwise cover your butt, it starts to look less like love. If, instead, you find yourself willing to grow, to admire the other person more than ever, to come up with whatever it might take to make it work, it starts to look more like love. I imagine there's a good deal of room to refine these criteria, but this is the general direction I'm inclined to look in.

Here are some of the things I have to consciously tell myself when I'm getting into a relationship. (1) Be yourself and do what feels right to you. If you have to censor yourself now, you'll have to do so in the relationship later, and that's no way to live. You need to have someone who accepts you for who you are. (2) Even though I want to spend all my time with her, I remember how bad I've felt in the past when I haven't kept up with friendships and activities that are important to me. I met this person when I was doing these things and the person was attracted to me, so I should still be attractive to them if I continue my activities. (3) I need to look at how I'm *really* feeling and not trick myself in to believing I feel otherwise. If I'm frightened or happy or sad or whatever, I need to acknowledge and deal with those feelings instead of masking or changing them so I look "right" to the other person. (4) Either we'll be compatible or we won't. The only way I'll know for sure is by being myself and seeing what happens. (5) Listen to your heart; it knows what the right thing to do is. (6) If I'm asked for some kind of decision and I don't know the answer, then it isn't the right time to make that decision. Wait until it feels right before giving an answer. Also sometimes not making a decision is a decision in and of itself.

————

Never underestimate the sexiness of danger. Being nice doesn't mean being boring—it should mean being unpredictable too. Like out of the blue sending flowers. Relationships need mystery to thrive—that includes being unobtainable from time to time!

————

I never sleep with someone I don't plan on being with for the long term. I don't sleep around partially because of pregnancy and disease factors, also (and most important) 'cause I equate sex with love and emotional attachment. If I sleep with you, I expect to be eating dinner with you every night. I expect to have you at Grammy's Xmas party, I expect you to adore me and send me "I'm thinking about you" e-mails.

————

There is something to be said about the chase, the pursuit being a very potent stimulus in romantic encounters. Knowing someone is head over heels for you in a way takes away some of the rush and buzz of the challenge, and unless you feel exactly as crazy for her, it can become off-putting rather quickly.

I'm always attracted to women who treat me like dirt, but I'm starting to realize that it's *me* who teaches them how to treat me badly. As long as I'm thinking that if I do enough "nice" things then I'll get the goods, I'm screwed. I'm not that nice.... Nobody is. That isn't the real me, and that's a turn-off. On the other hand, I've got a couple women right now who seem to be willing to do anything to be with me. I know I treat them disrespectfully and they don't deserve it, but it seems like their "neediness" brings out the worst in me. It's almost like they respect me too much so I compensate by respecting them too little. What's missing, in a word, is balance.

I've had an online relationship for almost a year and a half, and I wanted to meet him in person almost from the start. It sort of drove me nuts that he kept saying, "Some day, but not yet," but I knew my feelings were genuine and I felt he was worth the wait, however long. I was right. We met for the first time in May just for a few hours, which was probably good. We had lunch, went to a museum and to the zoo. It gave us each more of a feel for the other person. Since that initial meeting, there have been others ... and it's been wonderful. I realize now that he was looking out for the best interest of both of us in waiting, and that anything worth having *is* worth waiting for.

There's a difference between keeping secrets and maintaining privacy—two concepts that may have similar end results, but very different motivations. I think in any relationship there is a need for a certain level of privacy between the partners (whether it is romance, friendship, or whatever). When my husband and I first began chatting and developing our own online friendships, we shared a great deal with each other about various conversations and experiences. At first we both thought that we were being more "honest" that way. What we found was that we were being *too* honest, and it was interfering with our relationship. There was a bit of an adjustment period to get through, a bit of jealousy, but once we were over that hump and trusted this new online stuff, we learned to respect each other's privacy as well. Now we share general things about our various friendships, but we keep the details of our experiences private—all the involved relationships benefit from the privacy.

———

I want him to do nice things for me because he "loves me," not because he expects sex as a reward. If he is sweet, I do feel closer and the chance of him getting sex is better. It is not a game. When a woman feels loved she loves back in return. My mother called this "day-long lovemaking." However, there is not a woman who has not "given" her man sex when she didn't feel sexy, loved, or aroused. A man always knows when he wants sex. Not so with a woman. Sometimes we have to warm up to it. Sometimes we think we will like it and nothing happens. During those times I go ahead and finish even if I am not into it physically or emotionally. Sometimes we do it just because we love him. But don't say that because you did X or bought me Y, I owe you. That's the kind of stunts boys played in high school and college.

———

Crazy-making arises from trying to make all relationships meet some kind of conventional mold. Sometimes there simply isn't one. If you have a very special kind of connection, it doesn't have to be anything more than that. Make up your own rules to match the needs of the friendship as opposed to making the friendship match the rules of social convention. Enjoy it and take it as it comes.

———

Monogamy and Polyamory

Not many years ago, two people who lived together without legal marriage were considered to be "living in sin" and faced serious social censure. Now economics as well as preferences may dictate the makeup of any particular household—men, women, coupled, single. So also have both economics and personal preference allowed that the Judeo-Christian ideal of one woman and one man forever is not a style that appeals, or is even possible, for many. Relationships, like one-size-fits-all garments, do not.

My wife in many ways isn't enough. And I'm sure vice versa is also true. But I'm OK with her not being able to meet my every need, because frankly, I don't think that trying to fill *all* of one's needs is a worthwhile pursuit. However, an unending relationship with a woman who is willing to bear and help raise a family, be my friend, lover, cook, challenger, and the like, stick by me at the good and bad times, expect the same from me—that, to me, *is* a worthwhile pursuit. I'm not the most unselfish person on the globe, but I'm not a fan of selfishness either. I don't think there is a better environment for personal growth and childrearing than a monogamous marriage. It would be selfishness that would drive me to modify that institution. So, if at times I'm driven by curiosity to consider it, I take stock in what I have and what it has to offer—not just me but my family altogether—and just stay put.

———

One thing I enjoy about polyamory is that I can remain married and pursue other relationships as well. I do want to grow old with my wife, but don't feel it has to be in the context of being each other's one and only. Our relationship can change, and we don't have to see the loss of any one aspect of that as gone for the rest of our days together. We might no longer share something we did in the past, but we do have everything else. At the same time we can find that element in a different relationship, so we aren't losing anything.

———

I know some people who love each other in a noncommitted relationship because they both know a committed relationship wouldn't work for them. It's a *very* loving acknowledgment of each other. They know an exclusive relationship would be damaging to each of them and can continue to love each other because they don't have to commit to each other. They see each other when they can, and when they can't they can lovingly see that the other person is doing what they need to and isn't available. The connection is there even if they're apart.

———

Some will no doubt argue that if you're not actually having sex with someone other than your spouse you're still monogamous. Try telling that to my wife. Or try telling me. My cock may still be monogamous, but my heart's definitely polyamorous.

———

My husband and I are poly, and it was a long road to figuring out exactly what we wanted from our relationship and the relationships we might have with others.

———

I was scared, jealous, had mixed feelings about it all. I have overcome most of these feelings on one level, since we have actually had poly relationships with others. But, before we entered it, I was very uncertain.

———

I am a bisexual female, and I felt that it was important in my life to have the companionship of another female. It did not mean a completely sexual relationship, but rather a friendship that included sexuality. I think there is a difference.

———

My wife and I have been polyamorous for nine years together. We've been open since day one. When we met, I was involved with several different people simultaneously, and she was dating a couple. We've had multiple partners, both together and separately, over the years since. I known that jealousy is a common problem for people who are swingers or poly, but we haven't had any trouble with it at all. Not even once, in nine years. While it is never easy when a relationship dies (I was an emotional wreck when our ex-wife moved out, for example), we are better people for our lifestyle. I love watching another person fall in love with my wife, as it reminds me of all the reasons I did in the first place. We have learned much about ourselves through our interactions with other people, and we are a stronger whole as a result.

———

Poly relationships are different for all different people. You and your mate have to figure out what is right for you if you are to venture into this lifestyle. We found ourselves actually swinging at first (which is very different from poly relationships). We both knew that it was not what we were looking for. We were looking for the friendship, the love, the intimacy … for us this is what *poly* means. Since our realization and definition, we have found ourselves on a new path. We are more discriminating in finding a partner or partners. We are always redefining what we want in our relationship, which of course comes first, and then we try to figure out how the poly lifestyle fits into that. Sometimes we are not interested in pursuing anything at the moment, and there are other times where we are actively searching. I believe that the poly lifestyle is fluid, as I believe sexuality is. This means you must always keep an open mind and not be afraid of communicating with your partner(s). It is not a lifestyle for everyone, and it is also not an easy lifestyle. There is always something coming toward you that you have to deal with in one way or the other. Sometimes it is good, and other times it is not so good. I am still in the learning process myself.

———

For me, it really boils down to that I simply like to have more than one sexual partner in my life, *and* I happen to want a significant relationship with each person as well. I don't engage in sex with someone on a casual basis. There is something about this type of relationship that is fulfilling for me. It is hard to define. When I have another sexual partner, for some reason I become more sexual myself. My husband has even noticed this and obviously reaps the benefits.

———

Often when I talk to people about polyamory I am told that being with more than one person is just far too much *trouble.* Boy, don't I know about this trouble! But I also feel that much of the extraordinary effort it takes to establish and maintain multiple intimacies is due to the resistance (and often hostility) to non-monogamous arrangements inherent in our culture.

———

I think that non-monogamy allows people to form long-term relationships that can grow and change as the people in them change. They allow people to acknowledge and celebrate the connections they have with the people they love without ending the relationships when their growth moves them in opposite directions or causes them to be unable to fulfill their partner's needs.

———

I have been married for twenty-eight years. The first seven years I was monogamous, as was he. Then, for nearly the next ten years, we had an open marriage. Both of us had sex with others during that time, including a few encounters together with group sex (threesomes and foursomes) but mostly on a one-to-one basis. Part of it was out of curiosity, but most of it was for sexual pleasure. We closed our marriage back up when our son became a young teen, not wanting him to be hurt in any way by our outside play. There were other reasons, too. Lack of appropriate and/or desirable opportunity was a big factor. A change in the focus of our everyday lives was another. We also moved from a rural area in another part of our state to a suburban one close to a very large city, so our circumstances changed dramatically. I was too busy, for one thing, to even *think* about sex outside of my marriage. To be honest, there was a time then when I really didn't care about it at all, even in my marriage. My husband was also very busy, running a new business he bought and trying to establish himself in that role. He didn't seem to be very interested in sex, either. We both drifted away from it. Our circumstances have changed once again, slowly. My husband and I have an active sex life together again, and it is very satisfying. It has been like this now for more than a year. We do it more often now in a week than we did for a few years in a month! The truth is, I often think now that I would like to have sex with another.

————

A long time ago, early in our marriage, my husband told me that he will never be able to provide me with all of my needs. I came to accept that he and I cannot meet all of each other's needs in this life. I'd rather be realistic about that than let it destroy me, or him. I do love him very much, and he is my best friend. But I need other people in my life. In accepting that about myself and my marriage, I am open to feeling desire for someone else without it negatively affecting my relationship with my husband. I am also open to feeling love for another, in a very special way. That emotion does not take anything away from the love I feel for my husband or anyone else in my life. It lives and breathes as a separate entity of its own, one that makes me very happy. That is why I am considering having sex with one specific person outside my marriage. I'm not interested in swinging or swapping or group sex with strangers. My husband has mentioned recently being interested in pursuing sex again outside of our marriage on a very casual (and not routine) basis, but only with my approval. I have given that, with the understanding that he protect himself and me as well. I am not worried about his bringing home a disease nor becoming involved with someone in a way that would threaten my security, health, or well-being. So monogamy comes and goes in my life. I have been monogamous for nearly thirteen years and may or may not remain that way. I am open to the desire I have for another man now, because I will not shut myself off from life and my feelings again.

———

One of the hardest lessons I have had to absorb, being a polyamorist, is not taking troubles experienced with one partner along for a drag when I am with a second partner. It was the absolute worst thing to cope with when I was getting strong inklings that my very first poly love was not going to be associating with me for much longer. I wanted to chew the details over mentally whenever I could ... which obviously wasn't too great for making times with my husband intimate and loving. I am not certain how this tendency to get mired in feelings was worked through. It seems to have required almost a Zen attitude to do it.... I could do only what I could do (as far as letting the other fella know my feelings), and that should be enough to sustain my self-respect. It felt kind of cold-blooded at first, being so philosophical, but it did give me peace of mind, a useful perspective to latch on to ... but it takes some work.

Long-Distance Relationships

Once upon a time in song and story, young lovers vowed their love and devotion. Then he went off "to seek his fortune" while she waited chastely for him to return, fortune in hand, and claim her, often many years hence . . . and sometimes not at all. No letters, no phone calls, and certainly no e-mail. These days it's she who might be off to graduate school in another state as easily as his being reassigned by his company. Rarely can one simply pick up and follow, and if one does, it's not necessarily she who does it. It is almost a given that one or both partners in a couple have some work,

> study, or family obligation elsewhere, and these obliga-
> tions and the relationship are often in conflict. Some
> words on what makes a long distance relationship of any
> sort work . . . or not.

I've been in long-distance relationships, and they present a very different set of challenges than in-person relationships do. Erotic e-mail and phone sex are two ways of experiencing what you can with each other until you can be together, but those can be frustrating. All the explicit sex talk and heavy breathing can make you pine for your lover that much *more*. It's also important to realize that feelings can get very intense without reality to keep them in balance (as would be the case in person). I think in long-distance relationships, the most you can do is follow your heart and be honest with each other, and to take things one step at a time. Enjoy each letter and each phone call and have fun with your shared fantasies, but try not to let your emotions run too far ahead of reality. (I know that is much easier said than done.) The longer you wait to be together, the greater the chance that distance will interfere with the relationship you are building. You need to inject reality into your situation if you want this to be a long-term "real" relationship someday, so that the fantasies don't become the whole focus.

———

We would write daily journals and exchange them when we saw each other just to let each other know how we were feeling day to day when we were apart. We even made cassette recordings sometimes so we could hear each other's voices. But in particular, I'd spend the weeks dreaming up a setting and an idea for our next time together. Some romantic escape that would magnify our time together and make it easier to spend time apart.

———

Any sign from you—anything you can send—shows that you care. I was engaged to a woman who never sent me anything more than a postcard, and it broke my heart.

———

Any long-distance relationship is more fantasy than fact if the majority of the time you talk about what you're looking forward to instead of living today to its fullest.

———

Plane tickets, lots of plane tickets! Better yet learn to fly. Best still, move. I did all three! He was worth the effort. If your relationship is really meaningful, think about moving.

———

Care packages are wonderful. For example, when it became obvious that we were probably going to fall into bed very shortly after meeting, and when we discussed the necessity for HIV testing before we met, he sent me about six dental dams in the mail, with suggestions for use written in felt pen on each of them. Imagination can go a long way when you put together care packages!

———

My current marriage began as a 700-mile long-distance relationship. Our "dates" occurred about every four or five weeks. We kept it alive and "hot" with telephone conversations nightly, as well as first thing in the morning. We chatted often via IC. Within those two venues, we did enjoy phone and cybersex, as well as very long, deep conversations. It does take a bit of getting used to, but it worked for us.

———

FTD flowers? Why not? But don't send them only when she expects them. Send some because the day ended in a *y*. Send some because the sun rose after 4 A.M. Letters, handwritten, can help a great deal as well. Such a relationship can work, as evidenced by the rings on our respective fingers, but it is something that you both need to want deeply.

———

Probably the first thing was that we were devoted to each other, so there were no worries about 'others.' The next thing to do is get the cheapest phone rate possible. Letters and cards are nice, but don't expect them to be everyday events. Who's got the time? We always looked forward to visits. Plan something a little romantic a month in advance—then you'll both have something to look forward to. The week of my sweetie's visit my skin would be tingling from the anticipation! Sometimes my sweetie would send me packages. Crystal candle holders with my favorite scented candles, my fave flavor jelly beans, a CD he thought I'd enjoy . . . not real expensive, but it made me feel special to know that he would put thought into the gifts. I knew he was thinking about me.

———

Sooner or later, it's going to occur to her that she is missing out on a social life because of a spoken or implied commitment to you. She will subconsciously begin to resent you. You are probably passing up opportunities for involvement with other single women. This invariably breeds aggravation, frustration, suspicion, anxiety, and trouble. All this for a romance with less-than-favorable odds? If you do become involved in a long-distance relationship, don't forget—your fidelity does not ensure hers.

———

The more intensity there is in the long-distance romance, the higher the likelihood it will burn out. Keep it casual and friendly. Friendships by mail can last a long time, and who knows? Someday, circumstances may bring you together. It never hurts to keep your irons in the fire.

———

I carried on a long-distance relationship for more than a year with a fellow who lived five hours away—we've been married more than fourteen years now. Long-distance relationships, like any others, are deserving of priority time. When you are together, focus on each other as much as possible. When you're not together, stay in touch via phone calls, letters, or e-mail.

———

In my experience, if you've been in a serious relationship for at least a year and you're going to be apart for a year or less then it *can* work. My S.O. and I did it for one year. It helped that we had an end date when I would move out to be with him. We had been together for two and a half years and had lived together for three months when the long-distance shift came. We had talked about it beforehand, about his accepting a job in another state. I encouraged it.

———

Be very involved in life where you live. It will keep your mind off your separation. Another thing, use the computer to talk as much as possible. It's a lot cheaper than the phone.

———

There are all kinds of ways to make these relationships work. E-mail is great. If you have money (or are willing to give up other stuff for it), phone often, visit often, send presents and flowers and whatever is going to remind you that you are loved. Because relationships aren't just about kissing and going out. They're about feeling close to another person, and you can do that without being nearby.

CHAPTER 4

The Body

Have you ever had the pleasure of watching a two-year-old run around naked, shrieking with pure delight, or been tugged into the bathroom to be shown, with pride, what your toddler just deposited there? Too soon we learn that our body and its products are shameful, or smelly, or all wrong, (compared to models in the media), and receiving joy from the very same body can become problematic. We all sweat, burp, pass gas ... and we are all capable of intense peaks of passionate pleasure. Since the former comes with the territory, be sure you are doing all you can to get your fair share of the latter.

Getting Physical

When we speak of sex we usually mean giving and receiving pleasure with our bodies. Simple enough. Do what feels good, and refrain from doing what doesn't feel good. Would that it were that easy...

The key thing, I think, is to get comfortable with what you've got to work with. A woman who likes herself just the way she is exudes far more sexual appeal than one who is bummed out wishing she were bigger, smaller, firmer, or whatever. Besides, it's the size and firmness of the brain that really excites me, and there's no WonderHat on the market that I'm aware of.

I once had a boyfriend who was extremely self-conscious about his buttocks to the detriment of our otherwise enjoyable sex life. I tried to ask him about it gently, and even forced the issue at one point. As it turned out, he wasn't modest or ticklish. He had been traumatized by a childhood rape and a father who used to use a leather strap on his buttocks. Psychotherapy, a lot of hard work on his part, and a gentle approach on my part seemed to enable him to blossom. And you know what? His gorgeous buns look and feel better than ever to both of us. Moral of the story: He had to attain or regain intimacy and connection with his own buttocks before we could share them.

Sitting at a red light. Middle of downtown median strip construction zone. Four men, the first picks up a large, quite *heavy* brick and tosses it to the second, the second to the third, the third to the fourth, who places it where it is meant to go. They are in a rhythm, placing bricks. Such a simple thing, but oh so sensual. Watching the beauty of movement, the flex of muscle ... strength. You men are quite wonderful.

Hey, what's this noise about being fat? A bit of extra body can't hurt. I happen to think a girl can be pretty if she is fat too. It has nothing to do with the looks; it has to do with the appearance—how you behave around people.

———

Man, don't get me started on women's "I am overweight" issue. If a guy doesn't want to date you because the first impression he might have is "She is overweight, too much for me," you don't want to date him anyway! The person you want (and who wants you) is someone who sees *you*. Not your shell, not your clothes, not the car you drive, not your hair color, not your job, not your lipstick color, not the radio station you listen to. As long as you have self-confidence (and I know it can be hard sometimes) and aren't afraid of your weight issue, people will see who *you* really are regardless of what you look like.

———

From what I have gathered, a man can be apprehensive when a new partner is first formally introduced to his penis: "Will it measure up?" I equate this nervousness to that expressed by many of my female friends on what the guy will think of their naked body the first time he sees it. I find that I can be immediately put at ease about my body by a couple of sincere-sounding complimentary words.

Tastes

Do you swallow or spit? Is it a requirement of your satisfaction that your partner does? Woman or man, if you haven't ever tasted your own genital juices I strongly urge you to do so. Do they taste good to you? To your partner? Of course, what is a good taste is as debatable and individual as what a constitutes a good dinner.

Semen is alkaline. Acidic foods neutralize the alkalinity. Sweet foods "sweeten" or soften the unique flavor of semen. That's why pineapple juice works so well: it is very acidic and very sweet. Other sweet acid fruits and juices work too. A cup of juice at breakfast can make a big difference. Caffeine is alkaline and will make semen very bitter. Stop drinking caffeine. Too much red meat and dairy products can make semen taste bad.

———

Vegetarian men have the sweetest, mildest semen. Eat more fruits and veggies. Some things can make semen taste foul—asparagus and broccoli for some men. Pay attention to what you eat, and then note the taste of your semen to see if certain foods have a desired affect or an adverse affect. Drink water as your beverage of choice.

———

The best thing to sweeten semen is pineapple juice. Stay away from tobacco (good idea anyway), garlic, and asparagus (I don't care how good it is for you) if you want to help this process along. These can make your semen taste worse.

———

Try a little toothpaste on his member when you indulge. It sweetens the flow, and also acts as a little stimulant. (Not too much toothpaste; mild mouthwash works too.) A glass of wine next to the bed is very erotic.

———

Try offering him a steak early in the evening, provided you aren't vegetarian, of course! Red meat can remove the bitterness short-term, and acts as soon as it begins to be digested. This has worked for me and for several friends who experimented. Warmed chocolate smothered all over him can be neat too; just make sure it's not too hot.

———

I have only swallowed with one lover, and I think all of his various tastes are wonderful. I can tell when he's had spicy foods, or if he ate really light the day before, or if he's had a few beers, all by the way he tastes. The only time when his cum actually tastes bitter is when he's drunk way too much coffee.

————

Pineapple, kiwi, oranges, and most acidic fruits three days prior make secretions sweeter. Celery changes the taste. I have also found that abstaining from red meat for three days prior changes the taste. And what he drinks changes the taste.

Smells

There are multibillion-dollar industries manufacturing products to counteract the body's natural scents—deodorants, colognes, fragrance-enhanced shampoos, soaps, and sprays. Most humans enjoy caressing a fresh-from-the shower, squeaky-clean body. But vulvas do not naturally smell like flowers, nor armpits like peppermint. Most people also respond with pleasure to the natural sent of their lover's body.

I think smell and taste are two key things that tell whether or not a sexual relationship is going to work. Totally pheromones.

————

My husband's testes smell like a rich, fine, robust merlot. So much so, that I've never been able to drink a good red without thinking of him.

————

The fact of the matter is that some vaginas smell stronger than others. If you believe that your odor is excessive, I would reiterate the suggestion for a doctor visit. I travel a good bit and sit in meetings. As such, cotton panties really help me. Too, I wear pantyhose next to never, and when I must, I take them off ASAP. What I would not suggest is to try a bunch of sprays and powders (though I myself do use them during travel), but to shower at night and sleep without underwear. Douching might help. You may simply have to come to terms with the fact that you have a groovy-smelling pussy. There is a big difference between stink and smell.

———

I used to wear a coil for birth control, and I know this sometimes caused a pretty strong smell because of irritation. Medical treatment and the eventual removal of the coil cleared this up.

———

What I've found is that every woman smells and tastes different. Some are good, others are just plain odorous.

Body Hair

During the more than twenty years I have been a sex educator, hair has been a surprisingly hot topic—too much, too little, how to grow it, how to get rid of it. Rarely has the discussion been about what might be obvious—problem baldness. Occasionally it's about a preference for women with long hair—another topic you might think is a given—but not often. Far more frequent anxieties concern body hair or its lack. I never cease to be amazed at how much time and energy people put into its care, upkeep, and/or removal. Then I remember that high-born Egyptians used to have their slaves pluck out every emerged hair on their body every single day!

Do guys really care about this sort of thing? Some will, some won't. You'll find more opinions by guys on female body hair than you could ever imagine, ranging all the way from guys who prefer 100 percent hairy to 100 percent buzz cut.

———

The woman I had been dating for several months told me that before we slept together I had to shave all of my body hair. I couldn't believe my ears. We talked about it and I finally agreed—and am I glad I did. I am now such a convert that I think other couples should try it. We shave each other, which is a great prelude to lovemaking. The skin sensitivity after shaving really enhances sex. Just as I love the feel of her soft skin, she gets equal ecstasy from the feel of mine.

———

I prefer a nicely trimmed kitty. To me, a shaved woman looks much too young for me. I still find pubic hair on a woman to be extremely sexy. I love *Playboy* pics with a woman with her legs tightly together and only a small bit of pubes showing. To me, that's hot. I'm not into the *Hustler* (legs spread, lips spread) shots. My woman definitely better have hair down there!

———

Mine is shaved, but I don't do it. My husband does it for me. It's almost like a part of foreplay. We both enjoy how it feels when it's freshly shaven. He begged me when we first met to allow him to do it, and I was very hesitant. I mean, come on, how many people are comfortable with someone holding a razor to your most intimate parts? Remember, this was six weeks after we became intimate! I find it most relaxing now, and I'm the one begging for a shave.

———

I find body hair on a woman to be very attractive. I particularly don't like the artificial removal of pubic hair. While nipple hair is less common, it is still attractive to me.

———

This is to the woman who was concerned about health issues involved in shaving her pubes. I did it once or twice because my husband likes it. The main health problem was that the skin down there is very sensitive and seems conducive to ingrown hairs. These are very painful and can become infected. My solution is to shave with hair clippers on the shortest setting. This leaves about a quarter-inch of hair and precludes the ingrowth problem.

———

I appreciate a woman who is secure enough in her self image, and individualistic enough, that she cultivates a few things that make her different from her sisters. And I *like* a bit of female body hair myself. So for me personally, I would no doubt find a few hairs on a nice set of breasts to be a real turn on. It would be one of the neat things that makes you a special individual. *Vive la différence.*

———

I shave my puss because I find that it gives me heightened sensitivity, and my boyfriend certainly likes to give me more oral sex, which is definitely a plus! It isn't that bad shaving it if you sit in a bathtub full of warm water. The soak, the exfoliation, new razor every time—it all works.

———

I have found one natural beauty aid that surpasses any shave gel or foam known to humankind. It began when I was looking for herbal hair treatments, things to encourage a nice healthy gloss and increased hair growth. One bit of advice mentioned that a few drops of rosemary essential oil in a jojoba oil base would help. While looking this jojoba oil over, I read that it had multiple uses as a toiletry aid.... It conditions skin and hair, removes makeup, and so forth. The little one has no diaper rash problems since jojoba oil came on the scene. I tried smoothing some on in the shower for a bikini-line shave ... worked marvelously! I could see where to shave without foam to obscure the way, too. My skin was so soft afterward! I'm sold on it; forget shave gel.

———

Nair works wonderful, and every couple of days a hot bath or shower and a good razor to keep things smooth.

———

I have no pubic hair on my labia and bikini line and only maintain a small tuft just above my clit. I keep the tuft for purposes of decoration . . . different colors, for hanging beads from . . . that kind of thing. Sometimes I let the hair on my mons grow out so I can trim in different patterns or to shave completely off.

I am totally shaved and have been for about eighteen months. I really love it. I shave every night in the shower and use my electric shaver to get really close. I don't feel like a little girl, but instead feel very sexy. I can see everything and I love it that way. I love a man who will shave his scrotum and all around down there. I don't like hairy men and really find it discourages me from pleasing orally. If I make it nice for him. . . .

Nair works for me, every time, and all over.

Nair seems to irritate him. He has tried other lotions and creams as well, but they all do the same thing to him, so he sticks to the old razor.

Tried chemical removers once. My scrotum was just a little too sensitive. Stick with a good, clean, fresh razor and shaving gel. All you'll need is a little touchup every day or two. Your mileage may vary.

There is nothing like the feel of those smooth, freshly-shaven balls. I could stay there forever, just rubbing my nose, mouth, and cheek against them. Feeling them in my hands is a very lovely experience too. As for the pubic area, I like it trimmed down to about a quarter of an inch. I suppose the fact that I have been trimming down myself for half my life would have some bearing on my personal preference. I like it short because when I go down on my man I don't like to feel the tickle of hair on my nose, and I don't like to feel the hair in my mouth. And I can't say this enough. I *love* the feel of those smooth balls!

I like female pubic hair; among other things it provides a nice cushion during intercourse. I've had a few girlfriends who shaved it; it was vital for them to shave every day. Otherwise they quickly became uncomfortably prickly. In any case, why would a man want his woman to look like a little girl?

As a rule, I'd vote for neatly trimmed, but shaved is a nice way to surprise me on occasion.

I will take it either way. Hair, smooth, stubble, makes no never mind. I shaved once and the itch was incredible. And when it grows back those hairs are like spikes jamming into my skin. Plus I got ingrown hairs. I would never ask my honey to do anything I wouldn't, so we both sport beards. I haven't the time or patience to shave often enough. Hell, I can barely shave my face.

Personally I prefer women neatly trimmed, but not totally shaved. I like going down on a girl with hair. It just makes me want to lick and suck and taste her for a longer time. A shaved pussy does look nice but hair is just something I prefer.

I'm a guy who appreciates the "bare essentials," but it is not something I expect or beg for. It is great for a change. As for me, I shave regularly. At least once every couple of months. In the summer I don't shave as much, but stay "bald" most of the spring. I like the way it feels.

I prefer to be shaved! It makes everything so much more pleasurable for me . . . and also for him. Would you rather lick smooth skin or hairy skin? A no-brainer if you ask me! My boyfriend shaves also. I love it. He's the first guy that I have been with who shaves.

My former wife started shaving her pubic area, and I found it much easier to give her oral sex. I was able to breathe and stay down much longer, and try a few new things. Before she did this, I didn't think it made much of a difference, but I learned better. Around the same time, I tried shaving my pubic hair, but stopped for a while because the hair had helped me feel comfortable by keeping the various dangly parts from rubbing against each other. I haven't itched or pinched so much since before puberty. I've learned to live with the pinching, and I kind of like the smoothness of it all.

———

I have an alternative answer to the man who wanted to reduce the amount of hair around his penis. Although he wanted his scrotum clean shaven, he said he only wanted to trim the bush without undue discomfort. Like him, I don't want a bald area, just a little less hair. When I "simply trim the bush with scissors" the hairs become prickly and uncomfortable. Instead, what I do is burn some of the hairs off. I light an area with a match and blow the area before it reaches my skin. This leaves my hairs much shorter (but not baby bald), while also keeping them soft and comfortable.

Menstruation

Many religions teach that a woman is unclean once a month, nothing a righteous partner would want to mess with. While this taboo against intercourse during menses might make it even more attractive to those who enjoy flouting prohibitions, the truth is that blood-borne diseases like Hepatitis C or HIV can be more easily transmitted during menstruation. It's also important to remember that, although not as likely, a woman can still get pregnant while menstruating.

Sex at that time can be fantastic. Sometimes very little blood and others, very very wet, actually feels fantastic. Just put down a towel and go to town. When it's over hit the shower and hose it off. It's no big deal.

———

I've had some of the best sex at this time of the month. Every woman that I had sex with really enjoyed it. I have found that women are more sensitive when they are menstruating. Her hormones are going crazy, and she has more intense orgasms. I like it when she loses control. It does relieve painful cramping too.

———

My girlfriend says that her hormones make sex even more arousing during her period. The only thing that I find is that it's more slippery and wet during sex. I tend to like her tighter. But that's it. Blood is really no problem. I have found that every woman I've had sex with likes it during her period. Anything I can do to please!

Birth Control

Just as pleasure is a highly individual concept, what "works" as a method of birth control and/or disease prevention for any two people is not a universal given. I suggest that this issue be a part of any pre-sex conversation. Barring that, both men and women should always have handy a condom—or several—for any planned or unplanned heterosexual coitus. The Boy Scouts were right!

Regarding condoms—thinner does not always mean less strong or reliable, and the best are both. Lifestyles and Kimono seem to fit this category best. The traditional Trojan, on the other hand, feels like it is approaching kitchen rubber-glove thickness.

———

If a woman and her partner do not have latex allergies, condoms are very safe as a method of birth control. If they are used properly and in conjunction with a spermicidal foam or jelly, they are as effective in preventing pregnancy as the pill and give protection against STDs. And the pill has a number of contraindications that don't come with condoms, such as the risk of stroke. Many women, such as myself, have a very difficult time remembering to use the pill regularly. I got pregnant while I was on the pill for this reason. One cannot forget to use a condom, since it is a point-of-use method.

I've experimented with buying slightly larger condom brands, like Magnum and Beyond 7. The extra looseness at the head, with internal lube, can provide a little more friction.

The one trick to make a condom even bearable at all is to put lube on the inside, so that there is some sliding and a little friction around the head. I have never had spiritually meaningful intercourse with a condom (though I have had spiritually meaningful unprotected oral sex with the same exact women). The difference is cell-to-cell contact. For myself, I cannot have transcendent sexual intercourse with a condom. It has made me consider whether I should have condom-protected intercourse at all (in other words, hold off from intercourse until we can have unprotected sex safely). The reason is that it becomes too one-sided; my partner may be flying off in seventh heaven while I'm still earthbound; that's not fair to either of us.

Comfort is of course a relative term. Virtually all of the condoms on the market today can hold a football without breaking, but there are some variations on length and width available to most easily accommodate both the larger than average and smaller than average erection. Check *www.condomania.com* for a broad selection. All things considered, the Japanese lead the world in modern latex technology, with all kinds of high-tech additives to make condoms thinner and stronger than typical American brands. Kimono is a brand many men find especially nice. Swedish condoms in general are very good, and in the U.K. Durex makes a very complete line, including a broad line of flavored condoms for safe fellatio. Durex also makes the Avanti, the first polyurethane condom, which is a little less stretchy than latex, so they make them slightly larger. Some men really like them, as the plastic is non-allergenic and inherently slicker than latex, and the material transmits heat and tactile sensations better. It takes some experimentation to find what you like, but it's worth it. Remember the saying printed on the banana-flavored yellow condom I was given at a London pub—"Don't be silly, wrap that willy!"

———

My partner really enjoys Trojan Ultra Pleasure. He says they feel very thin and that they are not too tight. And they don't smell nearly as much as some others that we've tried.

———

I suggest the Avanti condoms. Those were the best I ever tried except those lambskin things. I just never could get over putting parts of a dead animal on my privates.

———

Avanti are stronger than latex (after being redesigned when breakage was a real issue), allow body heat to pass through, have no nasty latex taste and odor, and are unlubricated. Four-star rating from this condom hater. If ya gotta use one, make it as practical and unobtrusive as possible.

———

Every health class I've ever had says that if you use two condoms they will break because of the rubbing. This also goes for using a male condom and a female condom at the same time. I've never used a female condom, but it seems to me that they would be less likely to break because of their construction. My advice to you is stick to one condom and find a back-up method to use at the same time (diaphragm, sponge, pill) to be safe. It is scary when a condom breaks and there's no back-up.

———

If a condom breaks, the following can hardly be considered fail-safe, but it will at least give you something to do while you're waiting to get into a doctor's office. They also certainly won't hurt you. (1) Immediately douche with 1 ounce of vinegar in 1 liter of warm water. (2) Begin taking Vitamin C, 500 mg every hour until it produces loose stools. (3) Wash a stem of parsley and then insert it into the vagina for twenty-four hours. All of these actions will help to acidify the body, making implantation more difficult, but not impossible. It bears repeating: this is not a fail-safe method of birth control and should not be used as a substitute.

———

The kind of pill that I'm on I believe is the most common. It consists of twenty-one pills containing hormones, and seven pills that are just sugar pills. These don't do anything except help you remember to take your pill every day. The pill works by tricking your body into thinking it's already pregnant, thereby not releasing an egg to be fertilized. The seven days that you take the sugar pill, you will get a period. You do not need to use contraceptives during these seven days if you have been taking the pill correctly. If you don't want to get a period for any reason, such as going on holiday or a honeymoon, you can skip the sugar pills and go right on to the next pack of active pills.

———

The morning-after pill is most effective within forty-eight to seventy-two hours after the incident. Seventy-two hours would be the outside limit of effectiveness. It brings on a menstrual period to flush out the contents of the uterus before the fertilized egg implants in the lining of the uterus. It is not, therefore, an abortion-inducing pill, as some believe it is. Until the fertilized egg implants in the uterine lining, there is no pregnancy. The side effects may be heavy cramping, a heavy flow, and possibly nausea. In Canada, women are not able to keep a supply of pills on hand to use in case of condom breakage. They have to be prescribed by a physician or nurse practitioner.

Planned Parenthood would be able to help you if you can't get to an ER. But I wish that people who push the use of condoms for birth control would admit that condom failure is far more common than pill failure. Then women wouldn't find themselves in this kind of predicament.

———

My wife and I used the pill, but quit because of the health risks. We later found out the pill can cause a fertilized egg not to be implanted and thus expelled. We found this unacceptable. We now use Natural Family Planning; we monitor her body for fertility signs (temperature and mucus) and, if we want to avoid pregnancy, we avoid relations. In practice this means that we avoid relations for about ten days a month. After ten days of abstinence we are ready to go at it. At first I didn't like it, but it really brings back the feelings of love I had for her when we first dated. For us the abstinence period is a period of romance. For a reference on Natural Family Planning, look for a book called *The Art of Natural Family Planning*.

———

Many women using Depo-Provera, the injectable birth control, stop having periods.

———

Just over a year ago I began taking Depo-Provera, an injectable method of birth control. After experiencing just about every side effect known (and a few unknown), after a year I decided to go off it. The drug had totally killed my sex drive.

———

What I hated about Depo was the amount of weight I put on! I'm still fighting—no, I've quit!—I should still be fighting to take it off: twenty-five pounds!

Lubricants are not just an occasionally utilitarian requirement, replenishing what Nature has depleted, but can also be a sensuous adjunct to sex with self and other. As always in matters of personal pleasure, opinions vary widely.

My personal favorite lubes are Liquid Silk and, when something thicker is called for, Maximus. Both are made by the same British company. I love the feel of them—never sticky—and they don't use glycerin, which tends to exacerbate my tendency to get yeast infections.

———

I know one lube I'll never use again: ForPlay Watermelon flavor. It numbs you right up. Somebody's idea of funny, perhaps?

———

I tried a novelty lube this morning, ForPlay lube, watermelon flavor. It seems like a good choice when we bought it but in actual use it "numbed" my tongue and probably other areas as well. It wasn't supposed to be a topical anesthetic! I really liked the non-chemical flavor of ForPlay, but having my erogenous zones deadened verged on calamitous!

———

As far as numbing lubes, most contain very safe local anesthetics (like the variety found in Ambesol). Just be sure to read any warnings—some may not be safe to be consumed orally.

———

A couple of years ago, I surprised my S.O. with some of that stuff that heats up when you blow on it. I put some on his penis and went down on him. Within two minutes, he was totally numb and limp. He washed it off, but it was several minutes before the feeling came back and we were able to continue making love. We haven't tried that stuff again since.

———

Just be aware that Wet Platinum (and all silicone-based lubes) will do bad things to your silicone-based toys.

———

I have noticed a difference between lubes that are specifically for anal use and general purpose ones. Anal lubes tend to be thicker—a definite plus since the body is less likely to begin lubrication on its own as it might with vaginal stimulation. They may feel a little less natural than thinner lubes, but you really don't want anything getting dry while in the middle of the act.

Sexually Transmitted Dieases

For centuries society has kept people on the sexual straight and narrow with cautionary tales of unwanted pregnancies and public disgrace. Think of *The Scarlet Letter.* Times have changed, and for many, those fears have lost their hold. However, in these days of HIV and Hepatitis C, there are new bogeymen to keep us from free sexual expression. A popular TV star may flaunt his or her out-of-wedlock baby, but no one celebrates a debilitating illness. Be careful out there. Risk giving your heart, but do everything in your power to reduce the risks of transmitting your medical problems. The comments here are just a few snowflakes on the tip of the iceberg of a very important subject that no book on the topic of sexuality can afford to overlook.

To the woman who has been getting yeast infections from condoms with spermicide: It may not actually be the spermicide causing your "infections." I've done a lot of research due to my own difficulties. First I discovered that I was allergic to latex. My reaction was not unlike having a yeast infection. So I switched to non-latex condoms and then discovered that glycerin-based lubricant made me react too. I switched to silicone-based lube. Try different things to find what works for you.

When I picked up genital warts nine years ago, I thought my social and sexual life were going to end. The American Social Health Association and their newsletter *HPV News* were truly lifesavers for me. The newsletter offers medical and research updates and a lot of emotional support. (*www.ashastd.org* or 919-361-8425)

I have had genital herpes for ten years, and I get fewer outbreaks as time goes by. One technique I have found to minimize outbreaks is dietary. Arginine is in coffee, nuts, and chocolate and should be avoided, especially if you have the feeling that an outbreak is in the neighborhood. If a person with herpes feels a tingling, it's not too late to talk your body out of an outbreak. Lysine is in fish, milk, and potatoes, and if you took a supplement on top of these foods you would be that much better off. Four months ago I stopped drinking coffee and haven't had an outbreak since. Pay attention to your diet.

I want to thank you for printing information from a reader on how his or her herpes was treated. I immediately began taking Lysine and staying away from coffee and other agents that carry arginine, and I must say I haven't had an outbreak since.

When I met my fiancé three years ago he informed me he had herpes. We were always careful, but I ended up contracting them anyway. Needless to say I wasn't happy about it and he felt awful, but I hardly ever have breakout—and I wasn't angry with him. I took the risk myself. We take medication to help and now get a breakout maybe once a year. It's not great having this and definitely not healthy, but it's not a tragedy either. I wanted you to know that I did catch herpes while he didn't have a breakout

———

Ninety-five percent of urinary tract infections (UTIs) are caused by fecal material getting into the urethra. This can come from soiled underwear, not wiping properly from front to back, and also from vaginal intercourse after anal sex. A woman's anatomy may make her particularly susceptible to UTIs. Young children often get them from playing in a sandbox where cats have been. Other causes include the use of soaps or bubble baths. The onset of a UTI is rapid, within hours. I learned the hard way about deodorant soaps. Now I have a box of big-kid baby wipes in the bathroom.

———

I once had a really bad UTI. I got it from petting a cat that had a gum infection, after the cat licked her fur while cleaning herself. The doctor suggested that I touched my dick without washing my hands.

CHAPTER 5

Solo Sex

F ashion decrees everything from the height of a hemline to the year's preferred breast shape. The reputation of the act of masturbation also follows popular opinion. Some people remember when it was thought to be a sin, the cause and the result of insanity, a childish behavior, a perfectly acceptable private diversion, excellent preparation for partnered orgasm, and a healthy method of keeping personal plumbing in good working order.

I believe it was Woody Allen who said that one of the best things about having sex with yourself is that you don't have to dress up for it. Give thanks to Nature that the opportunity for anyone, male or female, child or adult, to enjoy a rush of gratification is always right at hand or available at the flick of a switch. One of the joys of being an adult is not having to ask permission from anyone. What a pity so much shame remains about giving oneself pleasure.

By yourself, you do not have the concern of pleasing a partner. It is all about you. Your mind is completely filled only with achieving your own pleasure. You know what you like best. You know how to bring yourself up, how long to hold off, and when to let go.

———

You might try having phone sex with someone while you masturbate. Just having someone to moan with can add nice variety to an otherwise solitary activity. Gives new meaning to the phrase "two heads are better than one."

———

Some very good tips on anal masturbation can be found at *www.very-koi.net/tutor/mast/mast09.htm.*

For Herself

Some females are lucky enough to discover in childhood how good it feels to ride a rocking horse or hump a favorite stuffed animal. All too soon we women are subjected to the notion that our genitals are so awful as to be nameless. While every other body part, major and minor, has a specific name, the essence of our womanhood was often referred to (if mentioned at all) as "down there." Products that disguise the "terrible" odor of our genitals and deal with the "unpleasant" fluids they emit are everywhere. It is not surprising that many women do not take pleasure in their genitals. Three cheers to those who have overcome some very negative messages in the name of personal power and satisfaction and have taken matters into their own hands.

I once used a mirror to watch my expressions while masturbating, and it was a memorable experience, rather like making love to another woman.

———

I have masturbated while others were in the office with me. To my knowledge they were never the wiser. These sessions would last a long time because I had to be very patient and tenacious in bringing about an orgasm since I couldn't use obvious techniques. Many times I would achieve orgasm by slowing and rhythmically pushing my clit down onto the hard folding chair I sometimes used when filing. They were very slight movements, ones that wouldn't call attention to themselves. It was hard wearing a poker face when I came though; I made sure I turned my face away from them. I'm sure I was flushed for a while as well. I often wondered if they ever caught the scent of my arousal and subsequent orgasm. They never said anything, so I assume they didn't.

———

As a teenager I often had painful menstrual cramps. When I married at age twenty my cramps decreased considerably, which I attributed to my system maturing and settling down. To my surprise, when I found myself partnerless in my mid-thirties, my painful menses returned. I put two and two together and began experimenting with masturbation as a "treatment." I've found almost total relief from menstrual cramps when I masturbate to orgasm. I have never heard or read of this method. Either I have made a great discovery (which I doubt), or our society's taboo against masturbation is so great that no doctor could ever bring him- or herself to recommend it.

––––––

It took me years to be comfortable enough to do this, but I now masturbate in bed with my husband sleeping beside me. Sometimes he knows I'm doing it and rolls over to help. Other times I'm sure he knows but doesn't let on, and sometimes he sleeps through it. (The other day he told me he woke up and thought the cat was on the bed licking because the bed was rocking! I took that as a compliment.) I sometimes lie so that my butt or leg is pressed against him. I find it very erotic to do it with him there.

––––––

I masturbate, and hubby knows it. He does, and I know it. Sometimes, we do it together; it is a fun addition to our sex lives. But we are pretty open about our sex lives, and tell each other what is pleasing to us.

––––––

I do it. However, it's only when my S.O. is not around. He's never expressed any particular interest in seeing, and I don't mind. I've only masturbated in front of someone once, and I could not climax with someone staring at me. I kind of felt put on the spot. It's like I'm too preoccupied with the distraction of someone else there.

––––––

Both my husband and I masturbate. Like many other women, I rarely climax during intercourse. I will often masturbate after he and I have had sex. He helps me by kissing and sucking on my breasts.

––––––

I have masturbated since preschool days. My partner does too, and we are both aware of it. For the most part we do it in private but on occasion I have asked him to do it in front of me and vice versa. At times I masturbate when we are making love if his attention is elsewhere!

———

I do it a lot more when I am not in a sexual relationship. If I am in a relationship where he is as sexually driven as I am, I very rarely do it. I am more likely to initiate sexual activity if I need release ... although if he is under the weather, tired, or not in the mood I am not afraid to ask him to hold me while I give myself an orgasm, which in many cases leads to a joint session. But if my partner is truly not up to it, I will do it privately so he doesn't feel like he is neglecting me or pressured to perform. I need clitoral or G-spot stimulation to have an orgasm and do not hesitate to touch myself during sex if he is unable or unwilling to do it. This has freaked out a couple of more conservative people, but I don't feel as if he is solely responsible for my orgasm. Besides, it enhances his pleasure if I climax during intercourse, especially if it is just at the point of no return or during his orgasm.

———

I've just recently found that if I keep the soles of my feet as flat as I can on the bed (and it's not that easy to do sometimes), it does something wonderful. I don't know why, something about the muscles that are used I guess.

———

Recently I had an experience with Dr. Bronner's peppermint liquid soap. The smell was great, and upon lathering up my body, I realized what a wonderful cool sensation it caused in my V. It felt *soooo* good, I found myself procrastinating getting out of the shower. I washed the same areas of my body over and over again. The feel of the hot water running down my body and the coolness in my V felt so amiable I ended up masturbating right there. Since that day on, I have been using this soap and going to work with a smile on my face.

———

I like to plan a long time, half an hour to an hour. Or, other times I need a quickie. I've got it down to a few minutes when I want it that bad. I rarely have a hard time climaxing. If I do, then I let it go and let the tension build up for a few days. Then I have a grand slam.

———

I'm a young woman in my teens. I used to do it every day, like seven to ten times a week or so, but now... once or twice a week.

———

When I'm not in a relationship I masturbate about every other day. Sometimes a few times a day for a few weeks out of the month. When I'm involved in a satisfying relationship, I rarely masturbate unless my lover and I are separated for more than several days. When involved I do love to mutually masturbate. But I'm usually so satisfied that I don't find any real need to masturbate alone.

For Himself

One of the first pieces of mail I received when I started writing my "Ask Isadora" column in the early 1980s was a twelve-page set of specifications, with carefully detailed drawings, of a masturbation device someone had fashioned for himself out of the cardboard center of a toilet paper roll lined with plastic wrap, fur, and all manner of others enhancements. I was, and still am, amazed at the ingenuity and creativity that someone (perhaps with too much time on his hands?) will display in the pursuit of pleasure!

I like to take long baths and recall (like a videotape) some of best and/or hottest lovemaking sessions with some of hottest lovers. I use liberal amounts of Vaseline, and sometimes baby oil. I never use *Playboy* or *Penthouse;* those woman are all fake. I actually look at a mag called *Naughty Neighbors.* If you are the type who wants to see pics of real women, few if any fake breast or plastic surgery types, this is an investment you should make!

———

I masturbate whenever I think about a girl's painted toes.

———

I do it every night and sometimes in the morning when I wake up. I also have my wife do it for me. Then it's really fun, because we do each other. Is it still masturbation when you do each other?

———

Masturbation is that creepy thing the Boy Scout book told me not to do, and the dictionary wouldn't tell me what it was. I *refuse* ever to masturbate again, but I *self-pleasure* typically once or twice a day (shower and/or bedtime) if not distracted by a current partner.

———

No point in a quickie for me. Not very satisfying, and I could come in less than a minute if I wanted to. I prefer taking it to the edge and holding it there as long as possible.

———

If an orgasm comes flying up out of the dark too soon, I almost always back off. I like to peak around two or three times—if I feel like really dragging it out, I throw in a mini-orgasm or two. My sessions usually run from three to twenty minutes once I start masturbating, depending on how early I want to get to sleep. I sometimes read erotica for an hour or two. Most of the time I do it just for the hormonal depressants that put me to sleep. Fortunately this habit hasn't led to trouble when in a more social sexual interaction.

———

I never use any lubrication when I masturbate. I don't have to use any. I don't know if that is the same with circumcised guys but I am European and still have the skin on the top of my penis. My way to masturbate is just by moving the skin up and down.

———

I have a smooth dildo with a large base that I like to insert in my anus. I use a harness to hold it in. Then I spend about forty-five minutes pumping up my penis. When it's nice and full I will spend about fifteen minutes bringing up head. I use Astroglide on the dildo and warm peanut oil in the pump. Time consuming? Yes. Worth it? Yes.

———

I sprayed my balls with hair spray one day. It was very cool and made them shrivel up. I came in minutes.

———

I do it pretty "cleanly"—little to clean up, just a quick handwash after I dispense with the tissue paper. Adding lube makes things considerably messier, though the added feeling can be pretty awesome. (When I do use lube, it's usually skin care lotion. Nothing scented.) Besides the messiness, another drawback to lubes is that they can really open up the pores, and the stinging can be a terrible torture. (Soap in shower—bad idea, past a certain point.)

———

Purchase one fat cucumber and a fat banana. Cut off one end of banana and squeeze all the pith out and save. Cut off one end of cuke and hollow it out, just big enough or a tad smaller than your dick. The cuke should be able to fit over entire shaft. Cut off the other end of the cuke, but not as far down, and save top. Place cuke onto and force down onto dick (might have to do some extra hollowing for a good fit). Place a teaspoon of banana pith into other end of cuke. Place little cap back on cuke upside down and place thumb on this. Stroke cuke up and down on dick for a suction-like grip put pressure on cap of cuke with your thumb. Apply more banana pith as needed. Guaranteed to feel as good if not better than some mechanical aids. Enjoy.

———

I am a man in my twenties. I masturbate nightly. If (due to trying to get fancy and failing) the orgasm was less than satisfactory, I usually come out of a light doze and go at it again. Almost always at night, unless I fall asleep before getting the deed done. Then it's taken care of in the morning . . . a rarity, though. So . . . between six and nine times a week. I'm not in a relationship, but when I was, it was probably between five and seven times a week.

———

Dry is nice; so is lubed. But let me say that until I learned how to have multiple orgasms all the masturbation I used to do was only a quarter as good. Now I have about five orgasms in about thirty minutes. Man, if I'd known then what I know now.

———

I wake up *every* morning hard as a rock. I jerk off on average three or four times a day, and in the past couple weeks I have been *soooooo* incredibly horny it's more like six times a day and yet . . . I have *never* had a wet dream!

———

We all have our fantasies, and they sometimes change depending upon our mood. When you are alone and masturbating you can be anyone you want, you can dream anything you want and pretend to be with anyone you want. I fantasize a lot, and although my fantasies are very vivid, they usually end abruptly when I come . . . but nothing is wrong with a good fantasy!

———

Extremely good lubrication, quiet place, good-quality nude pictures that you can mess up, and changing hands in between; yeah, those are some very simple and very good ingredients I've discovered through personal experience.

———

The best way I've found to masturbate: Index finger on the frenulum, on the underside of the penis right below the head, through my foreskin, rubbing very slowly and with meditative concentration, on my side with legs together. Feels wonderful, takes a long time, and the orgasm is incredibly detailed and intense.

———

Bring yourself close to orgasm and back off. Do this several times (takes some willpower); maybe use a clock and set a minimum amount of time (ten minutes, whatever) before which you are not to orgasm. This teasing usually intensifies the orgasm when it finally arrives.

———

Try unclenching all those muscles in the floor of your pelvis as you get close to orgasm. You'll probably drop quite a few levels in arousal, but if you do this close enough to orgasm you're probably in for a treat. I just recently started trying this out—and it's a hell of a lot harder than it sounds to get to orgasm as well as keep those muscles relaxed. They want to clench right back up, and they will if you don't concentrate on keeping them relaxed. If you manage to get past the point-of-no-return and keep those muscles relaxed for as long as you can, that first throb of orgasm will just stall out—that falling, yawning sensation right before the ejaculatory spasms begin—will last for a while.

———

Stroke to orgasm any way you want to, but as soon as you get past the point-of-no-return, stop touching yourself completely and ride out the (weakened) orgasm on autopilot. When you feel the last spasm coming (you do have a good idea of about how many spasms you have during orgasm, yes?), start stroking again, and make a mental effort to think erotic things. In less than ten seconds, another point-of-no-return will hit. You can keep stroking for a full, strong orgasm, or repeat this process and ride out a second orgasm . . . and a third . . . and a fourth. I got up to five once. This is a little hard to master, and timing can be messed up. But I find, since the orgasm caused by a mistimed stroke is small and weak, the refractory period is significantly smaller. I hope it's the same for you.

———

Resist the urge to stroke faster during orgasm, and try to keep it under one stroke a second (I think we usually average something on the order of three strokes a second or more during orgasm and right before). This really draws out the orgasm, deepens it.

———

I love to masturbate and I love to do it inside and out.... Nothing beats a good jerking off alone out in the great outdoors!

———

I believe *autofellatio* is the technical term. Thirty years and fifty pounds ago I would take a hot bath, relaxing in the steaming water. One can bend and stretch much more after a warm bath. When everyone was gone from the house, I lay totally naked on a soft rug, with my head near a heavy sofa or near a counter in the family room. I could easily bend my legs back over my head and catch them under the sofa or under the edge of the base of the counter cabinet. Once my feet were secure over my head, I could curl up and take my own cock into my mouth. In retrospect, it was not much of a blow job, but I could explore the head with my tongue, swirling it around, and tasting my own pre-cum. Once I had stretched out and curled up, I could usually release my legs, sit upright, and resume this position. I don't really remember ejaculating in my mouth, although I suspect I did. Although I could barely stretch to get to near the base (I'm just average, neither big nor small in endowment), I enjoyed the sensations. My sense is that this was essentially masturbation of the head of my penis by my tongue. I could not move up and down the shaft rapidly like a more conventional blow job.

———

I have been able to bend myself enough to take the head of my penis in my mouth. I had done it a couple of times in my teens, and even came in my mouth. For me, being average in size, I couldn't take the whole thing in, just the head. What I did was apply suction to pull the head in and out of my mouth. With some assistance from my hand, it felt good enough that I actually climaxed. Actually? Hell, it felt great!

———

A few years ago I developed an unusual masturbation technique that other men might also enjoy. I usually lie on my back with my knees pulled up toward my chest. When my penis is semi-erect and still quite flexible, I press it back between my legs and gradually push it inside my anus. Once I have a couple of inches engulfed in my anus I then use my hand to slide it in and out until I reach orgasm. It takes some coordination, but it's actually easier than I thought it would be. Having anal intercourse with myself, being both active and receptive at the same time, feels very satisfying, sensual, and exciting.

———

I fail to understand the fascination with masturbating by placing one's penis up one's ass and rocking back and forth. This form of masturbation is commonplace in Europe. It originated in Italy and is commonly referred to as a *stromboli*—sausage in buns. Not to take any offense at your column that called us twisters, pullers, and pokers; we prefer to be called "strombolists." There are more of us around than you think.

For Your Partner

There are exhibitionists and voyeurs of both sexes, grown-up kids who still like to play doctor (some of whom *are* doctors!), and those who simply learn best by seeing certain kinds of touches in action. Entertainment or education, masturbation can be more than an act of solo gratification. Because masturbation is still an extremely private act, some are titillated by the taboo of watching another person do it. This sharing of a most secret act can be perceived as proof of profound intimacy. Whatever your reason, two people can play grown-up Show and Tell to their hearts' desire.

I do it, and have done it in front of a lover. My previous lovers did, and I always asked them to do it for me, because it excites me and I want to learn what they do to give themselves pleasure.

———

I think that a guy jerking off while looking at me is one of the best compliments that he can give me. I get very turned on by watching a guy touch himself and giving himself pleasure. I would have no problem with any guy doing that and, I must admit, I enjoy it.

———

I'm very happy that my hubby is so comfortable around me sexually that he can feel free to casually masturbate in my presence in response to something he feels erotically aroused by ... be it a sexy actress or model, a fantasy he's recalling, or the stock reports on CNN! We're both very sensual creatures and it really excites me! Sometimes he invites me to join in, and I'm more than eager to oblige him, but he does it so often (not to climax usually ... it seems just for mood enhancement) that I've come to accept it as the norm. I quietly enjoy basking in the warm glow seeing him so happy gives me!

———

My boyfriend told me he could suck himself off. The idea was both fascinating and arousing to me. I convinced him to do it while I watched. He can, indeed, at age thirty-eight and not in ideal physical shape, manage to give himself head. He positioned himself on the bed with his back against the headboard and brought his feet over his head to the bed. In this position, it was possible for him to take the head of his penis in his mouth and suck and stimulate it enough to reach climax. He says he does this much less regularly now, as it pulls on the muscles in his neck and back, but when he was younger, he did this with some regularity. Now, he has me, and as much as it is nice to be able to perform this act upon himself in a pinch, he prefers to lie back and enjoy what I can do for him. I must admit it was quite a turn-on to watch, though!

———

My husband uses nothing when he masturbates (he is circumcised); on the other hand (ahem), when I play with him, we end up using hand or body lotion. It takes me a lot longer to get him to climax than one of his do-it-to-yourself ones. He tells me it's because he *knows* how to touch and what pressure to use to achieve an orgasm. At least he doesn't seem too upset when I approach him with a handful of lotion, as long as I've warmed it up a little prior to application.

———

I am intrigued by female masturbation. I would love to watch a woman pleasuring herself. I would find watching her every move, what she does, where she touches herself, the rhythm, the movement, how her pace changes at different peaks. That way I could imitate when I go down on her. I would find it very . . . educational. But I have yet to have a GF that was interested in doing this for us.

———

I love to watch and be watched. It is a very trusting and intimate thing. I have a fantasy of doing it for someone I barely know at her request! The idea really turns me on!

———

Mutual masturbation is highly recommended, especially when you are getting to know one another. How would he know how to give me an orgasm if I didn't first show him? Of course, he wasn't too difficult to figure out, but I learned a lot by watching anyway.

CHAPTER 6

Outercourse

There's no doubt about the definition of sexual intercourse—penis enters, is engulfed, then moves in and out. For some folks that's the be-all and end-all of any sexual interaction, the definition of sex itself. For some, all the other lovely touching, licking, nibbling, gazing is equally if not more important. The "other" is not *foreplay* any more than salad is an appetizer. Both salad and foreplay can be before the main meal, after the main meal, or the main meal itself. We used to call all this stuff "necking and petting," and I think it was more enjoyable as a longed-for happening in itself than as a perfunctory step in a familiar routine. Sex need not be a construction project: "Fit prong A into slot B after two minutes of pressing on area C." Think more in terms of a Treasure Hunt with prizes given for creativity as well as discovery.

Sex Play

I am often asked what the secret of being a good lover is, as if the questioner knew there must be one and he or she were absent from class the day it was revealed. Actually, if there is one thing that makes a man or a woman almost universally appreciated as a sex partner—as a *pleasure* partner—it is the quality of attention paid. Gather information with your lips, fingertips, eyes, ears, even your toes. Register a partner's response to what you are doing and act on that. Smiles, sighs, eyelash flutters, skin warmth, dampness, all tell their own story. It also helps dramatically if you abandon all scripts about how it's supposed to be and improvise according to the mood of the moment.

I make no distinction between foreplay, sex, afterplay, cuddling; it is all lovemaking to me. One blends into and out of the other in no particular order. There is no dividing line. Foreplay is an abstracted and mechanistic description that has no meaning in my view of sex.

Any slow, deliberate touch feels fantastic! Sprinkle in some kisses and even a gentle bite or two ... and I am ready for whatever he'd like to do next. I find the inclusion of toys like the feather duster from the Kama Sutra honey dust canister or a fine paintbrush tracing patterns on the skin to be *really* pulse-quickening. It may be unusual to like both bites and the feel of beard stubble on my ass, but it is a very keen way of arousing me. I love the word *ass*.... It has something lusty, terse, and direct about it. One of those words you can manage to say when your civilized veneer is peeled away by carnality.

Can you please give a clue to the men who complain that their wives or girlfriends aren't into sex? Maybe we women need more than we're getting. A blow job may be foreplay for them, but not always for us. When we're not lubricated it may be that nothing has aroused us, not because we're not interested. More simple touching, kissing, and "I love you" every once in a while would work wonders. And, slow down, men. Sex should be an experience, not a race toward orgasm.

———

If a woman is submissive, I get the feeling that she is just doing it because I want to. What I want is for my lover to want me back, and to demonstrate it by being assertive enough to let me know, whether it's by taking the first step, or if I make the first move, she can grab my shirt, pull me to her, and say, "Yeah, you bet!" I love it when a lover tells me what she wants . . . and on occasion *demands* it.

———

When I'm giving my Dearly Beloved a hand job, I find positioning is important. Usually he lies down on the bed and I scooch up to his left side, my left leg extended under his body and the other leg curled between the two of us. This allows me to stroke him with my right hand while using the left hand to play with other areas. It really takes time to learn how to touch. This requires lots of experience, experimentation, and feedback from your partner. In the past I was probably too firm, or not firm enough. Now I can adjust my firmness to his benefit—a bit firmer for more stimulation, easing off for teasing benefits as he gets closer to orgasm. I often begin by gently squeezing his cock in my hand, and then slowly stroking him into a full hard-on. I find it works best if the finger or thumb on his cock completely follows through on the stroke—that is, *over* and then *past* the sensitive spot on the underside of his head. I vary the strokes between fast and slow, interspersed by some squeezing. Above all, I pay close attention to his responses so I know what to do next. While the right hand is busy I cup his testes in my left, giving them a gentle squeeze or caressing them lightly. Sometimes I'll cup them and gently press them upward as I continue to stroke him. I'll also apply a bit of pressure to his perineum as he's approaching orgasm, this stimulates the prostate and he finds it highly enjoyable. Those who are so inclined can also incorporate anal play into this position. A bit of oil or powder can be used to ensure a smooth stroke. We usually don't use them because from time to time I might want to lean over and take him into my mouth as a bit of added stimulation.

The best response I have gotten is when I use my mouth in conjunction with the hand motion. Keep your mouth around the penis and go up and down with your hand. The biggest problem I think women have is getting tired. Men are used to this jerking off motion; women are not. I try to switch hands a lot to keep from getting fatigued.

My S.O.'s ears are way too sensitive for much tongue-play. He can only stand a couple nibbles or a quick lick. He says it is like a high-voltage shock going through his body. I, on the other hand, *love* to have my ears smooched, licked, and nibbled on. It sends such fantastic tingles straight to my clit. I could orgasm quite easily with a skilled ear nibbler.

I will melt at the slightest hint of ear nuzzling! For me it is the warmth of his tongue and the sounds it makes, you know the kind of sound I am talking about, those wet, moist, slurp ... noises, the noises that sound like sex! Purrrrrrr.

Sex is all about the intimacy that you are sharing with the person you are with. Having a mirror there would just take attention away from the other person, so I guess I'd have to give mirrors a big thumbs-down.

To do this, you'll need a sable artist's brush, about as big around as your pinky finger, and some warm oil. Almond is especially nice. Some scented candles in the room and sensual music will contribute to the hedonistic luxury of the evening. Begin by inviting your beloved to a sensual massage. A fondue pot in its frame, set above a tea light, will keep the oil warm throughout the process. Towels can be spread on the bed if you're concerned about staining the sheets. Rub the oil into your beloved's body: back, breasts, buttocks, legs, shoulders, until she's glowing and sighing with contentment. Have her roll onto her back and use whatever means you normally use to rev the sexual engines. When she's nicely primed, have her open her legs. Here's where the paintbrush comes in.... [Note: Discreetly test the temperature of the oil on your wrist before you begin.] Dip the brush in the warm oil and use it to trace along her body—it will feel like a delicate, warm tongue. Work tiny O's of delight around her nipples and down her belly ... into the navel and continuing downward. Use broader strokes up the insides of the thighs and the bottom of her cheeks. Delicately flay the rosebud of her anus if you think she'll enjoy it. Dip the brush in the oil often to keep it wet and warm. Use the brush to "lick" long strokes against the interior and exterior of her labia. Keep your touch light throughout, but not too light—the flaying out of the bristles can help guide you. Spread her labia to expose her nirvana. Use the brush to trace the ridge of flesh, from where it blossoms from her mound to the very tip. Trace down the length of one side of the ridge, then the other. Work small swirls of pleasure around the tip, alternating with longer strokes along the hood. If you look closely, you'll see the exposed tip of the clitoris. Some woman love to have it stimulated directly, others find the sensation too intense. Experiment and conduct yourself accordingly. Take your time (a long time) and keep it up, until her hips are bucking. This is an excellent introduction to oral pleasures for those who wish to experience it, or those who want to learn more about the exact manner in which to please their partners. She'll thank you for it.

———

One cannot go wrong in playing with my ass. There is no wrong way to play. (I especially love when he plays with my ass through silky pajamas.) One small hint: As with the breasts—the crease underneath the ass (or breasts, as it were) needs more attention than it currently gets, in my opinion.

———

I absolutely love having my butt squeezed when I am being kissed. It sends shivers throughout my body.

———

Having my ass kneaded and squeezed is nice, but I prefer to be spanked now and again between passionate fondles!

———

When my lover and I have sex, *the* single most erotic part of it is to watch my lover's face as her arousal builds and finally while she comes. My lover knows this, and even if her eyes are not open or if I am thrusting her from behind—she will turn her face so I can watch her come. To me that is the most intimate image a lover can share with me—to let me watch her face while she comes. If her eyes are open— so much the better—but even if she is lost in her own orgasm—I enjoy it and the sight quickly brings me to orgasm too. Funny, often while we are together in a group and I am watching her talk, laugh, and interact with friends, I'll get a little jolt of excitement knowing that I can picture in my mind at any time the vision of her head thrust back—neck exposed, mouth open—coming.

———

When my boyfriend and I first started having sex, we always did it on the bed. A total of thirteen times on the bed and no orgasms for me. We used the floor out of necessity one night and—*bam!* —I got one! We never use the bed anymore, and we always joke that when we move in together all we need is a place with a lot of floor space. Perhaps the floor is better because it is harder and offers the guy more ability to control his actions. Doesn't hurt to give it a try though. Lord knows I have had the best with the floor!

———

I have a few rules about sex . Rule number 1: If we can't talk about sex, we shouldn't be having it. Rule number 2: Coming is not a requisite for good sex. Rule number 3: If he doesn't give oral sex, I don't either. This is evolving into: If he doesn't give oral sex, he's history.

Are we so perfectionist-oriented now that we feel we really only have one shot to impress someone sexually, so we go all out planning the first time? God, I hope not, or I wouldn't even be in a relationship right now! I was a total disaster the first time with my S.O. I thought "foreplay" was something golfers did. I thought "responsiveness" was something you looking for in a good steering wheel. And to make it worse, I didn't think anything was wrong with my style! Oy! Thank God some people out there are willing to teach people a thing or two before resigning them to the scrap heap of sexual history.

My hair is shorter than short now, but once upon a time I had long, long hair. Straight and very fine. I wrapped it around an ex's cock and stroked him to a very nice orgasm that way. He loved it. We tried a silk scarf later but he said the hair felt better.

Though I'm not generally of a submissive bent, I enjoy being blindfolded and restrained for fellatio. What I like better than feathers are those thick brushes for applying makeup with say a jar of powdered sugar. I love being surprised with differing sensations, like alternating between ice and hot candies.

I've always had a soft spot for women's necks, and women who neck, and women who kiss necks. A light touch of nails on the back of my neck as I dance slow and close with a woman is an incredible turn-on for me. I think the neck is highly underrated as an erogenous zone. I have a friend who says the most intense orgasm she ever experienced was located in the side of her neck. Ever see classy Japanese nude portraits? The neck gets more attention than breasts do.

God, do I love foreplay! Do you realize, as men, how infrequently we touch another human being, and how infrequently we are touched as well? When human beings touch each other (and it's the good, desired kind), all sorts of neat, fun, warm, endorphin-type hormones are released. As a result, all sorts of emotional bonds tend to be formed. As men in American society, from the age of twelve or so to the time we actually have sexual partners (and for some of us, that's a decade or so), we have no intimate contact with other human beings. No hugs, not a solitary back rub, nothing. A haircut is as close as we get to an erotic experience. A human baby that is left in a crib and is never touched will grow up to be maladjusted and antisocial. Perhaps that has something to do with why teenaged boys have so many emotional problems (well, aside from more testosterone than any sane human being would know what to do with). So when the time comes for foreplay, it's a thing to be savored, experienced, recorded in our minds for those lean times that may come. In the process, it also feels damn good to make another person happy. Makes me feel useful and wanted. Intercourse is just one aspect of human sexuality. The rest, foreplay, constitutes the majority of things we can do for each other.

———

Funny thing is, I have actually run into a woman who could not care less about foreplay or taking it slow. She confessed to me that she preferred to be taken, hard and fast, and to get it over with. This was honestly one of the most shocking and disturbing things I ever heard in my life.

———

My ex started out as an amazing lover ... always taking lots of time for foreplay. He'd start out with long erotic kisses and when the kissing warmed us up, he'd move down to my breasts, then he'd move down.... Now he just kisses me a couple times, skips the breasts, goes straight for the oral (only to make sure it's well lubricated), then tries to stick it in. And that's if I'm lucky. For whatever reason, he figured he didn't have to do all that work anymore. A woman *needs* to be warmed up . . . unless she is already there from other sources. A man needs only to have a hard-on and he's ready to go.

I know that I derive just as much pleasure from foreplay as my lover does. The idea that what I am doing could bring her that much pleasure is the most exciting thing in the world to me. I just can't imagine anyone not wanting to give as much as they get!

For me foreplay is *way better* than the act of intercourse. Nothing beats watching your lady come and watching to see just how horny you can get her.

I couldn't care less about any foreplay that is aimed at pleasing a woman. I spend time kissing and nibbling on my wife's ears, neck, shoulders, arms, wrists, licking her hands and gently sucking her fingers, tracing my tongue up her side and around her breasts, slowly, very, very slowly centering in on her nipples and then licking, sucking, and nibbling them before moving on. From there I move my tongue, while my hands continue to gently and lightly tickle, down across her stomach and across her hips where I stop to nibble on her hip bones and watch her get excited and jump from it. Continuing along her inner thigh, I come extremely close to her labia and tempt her with my warm breath, on down to the back of her knee and along her calf, stopping at her foot. Here I can lick her instep and watch her squirm because it tickles, or nibble with just the right amount of pressure to make her pleased at the touch. Then I again begin my ascent, tracing a new path on her other leg to her luscious lips. Here, I can and will probe her outer and inner lips and clitoris with my tongue, fingers, and face for as long as she will allow me. *None* of this, however, is aimed at pleasing her. It pleases me.

Have your partner thrust a couple of fingers or a toy inside you as he sucks your clitoris. Have him continue to suck after your orgasm . . .

keeping you on the edge of where it's so sensitive it almost hurts ... but still feels good, too. This takes practice and trust. He can watch you for signs that it's becoming too intense and then back off for a few seconds. Have him insert a finger and continue to rhythmically stroke your G-Spot after you come. He can keep you at a blissful level for a half-hour or more. He may need to occasionally stimulate your clitoris, too, to keep you at a level you like.

A good kisser is a joy forever. And the great thing is, you can kiss in public and not get arrested for it, unlike so many other sensual acts. Matter of fact, I like kissing so much that it's a key element for me in gauging possible sexual compatibility with a woman.

Sometimes when we're in the mood and we're driving, she'll reach over (no matter who's the driver) and give me a slow, easy hand job to get us both good and horny, but I could never come from a hand job. It feels good, don't get me wrong, but orgasming or coming is out of the question. My body is too used to my own hand being down there.

One of the best things about a hand job is how close you can be with each other. One of my favorite things to do is to lie next to my lover, with my arm under her neck, her head on my shoulder, and watch her face as I bring her off with my fingers. If she is giving me a hand job at the same time, it can be similar to a 69 in that we are pleasuring each other at the same time. You just can't beat the intimacy of the eye contact, watching the changes in expression as your lover goes through all the different phases of arousal, and watching their face when they climax is just the sexiest thing in the world. Just a different way of doing things that adds variety to life and love.

Nipples and Breasts

Women's breasts, and nipples particularly, are given major coverage as sexual playthings in our culture, but not too much is heard about men's. Many men wake up to the erotic potential of their own nipples late in life only because of the attentions of a creative sexual partner. Any discoveries to be made in your life?

There's a wire that runs right from the very tip of my nips to the very tip of my penis. Suck on one and the other gets hard.

———

I think it's possible to develop one's own erogenous zones over time. When I was in my mid-twenties, I would've said that my nipples were not much of an erogenous zone; now they're one of the most sexually sensitive areas of my body. I've also been with several women who loved having their necks kissed and at least one who loved kissing mine. The fact that she was so into it was highly stimulating mentally and emotionally.

———

There can *never* be enough smelling, licking, kissing, stroking of the underside crease of the breast between breast and rib cage. That is probably the most sensitive spot on my chest, and I love any and all attention given there. Kneading and squeezing of my breasts is almost always too much. I'll pass. I don't know about others, but my breasts bruise easily. Too much sucking and I've got a hickey for a week. Too much squeezing, the same. So, go down and play underneath—I'll never stop you, but please, don't squeeze my Charmins.

———

The woman lies on her back straddled by the man, who places his erect penis between her breasts. One party or the other squeezes the breasts together to close around the penis. The man begins thrusting motions between her tits. Depending on the length of his strokes and other size relationships, she may be able to lick the head of his penis on the forward stroke. When the man reaches his climax, the woman may wind up with a pearl necklace. This is one of our various forms of outercourse.

———

Pearl necklace is lots of fun and gives enjoyment to both the giver and the receiver. You start by lubing up the breasts and then push them together and slip your cock between the breasts. Then you proceed to thrust yourself between them. As your cock pops out the top of the breasts, your partner can catch it in her mouth depending on the position you're doing this in. When you come, it is all over her breasts, neck, and face. Then you can either spread it around or clean it off. It depends on how you and your partner feel about your cum.

———

My nipples are one of my favorite erogenous zones. I like to go from a light touch of the finger and tongue to having them mildly pinched. Your mouth and tongue can become your partner's best friends: light licking, sucking, circling the nipple, light biting.... I suggest *light* biting at first, because you want to work up from there to find your partner's limits.

———

The best action is nipple-to-nipple action. Take your shirt off. Oil up your nipples and place against his. Rub like crazy.

———

In the past few years my nipples have become incredibly sensitive; even the seat belt can get me horny. I am a man who gets incredibly turned on by having my nipples rubbed. I like to start out having them rubbed through my shirt; the tell-tale sign is that you can feel the little bumps. When they are hard like that, then you know I'm feeling it! When my shirt is off, just gently rubbing them back and forth is usually the best, but to really get me going, lie beside me and take one nipple into your mouth and lick it back and forth while rubbing the other with your hand. Occasionally drop your free hand to my balls and rub your hand up my shaft and return to the nipple, all the while licking the other one.

———

My S.O. just loves to have his nipples pinched hard. I roll them firmly between my fingers, but most of all he likes me to bite them and lick them. I also suck at them.

———

My preference is for clothespins; but I think those might be a bit much for some. I mention them because they may be found around anyone's house and it might be worth an experiment. If you like them, you can, as I have, buy black rubber-tipped clothespins or stainless steel clothespins. The kind to look for are those with an adjustable threaded screw on the side. It allows you to set the tension. And you want to be sure that they come with rubber tips covering the metal. If you find these too soft, you can change the tension or remove the rubber tips.

———

Pierced nipples = more sensitive nipples? My case, yes, absolutely. Went from little sensitivity to much sensitivity. In addition they physically grew significantly.

———

The nipples of a friend of mine aren't particularly erotically sensitive, but kissing and nibbling her neck affects her the way nipple-work does most women. She doesn't mind if you suck on her nipples, if that turns you on, but it doesn't do anything for *her*.

———

My boyfriend did something that surprised me because it seemed really obvious but no one had done it before. He paid attention to the whole breast and not just the nipple! Wheeeee! Personal revelation that I'm not just some kind of sucking toy. He bit his way around the side.

———

It depends on how sensitive my breasts are at that moment, but a lot of kissing is always good, touching lightly on the sides of my breasts through clothing first, then as the clothing comes off, more light touching and stroking the whole breast prior to using his mouth. As things get more intense, sucking on one nipple while playing with the other breast is wonderful. I've had a lover almost bring me to orgasm just from this.

Sex Talk

Elsewhere in this book are included comments on sex and the senses of sight, smell, and taste. And, of course, the sense of touch is a major part of what sex is about. Hearing as an erotic sense is often overlooked. The sound of a person's voice may be a factor in initial sexual attraction, the right kind of music can create desire, the "night music" of lovers' bedtime moans and gasps can spur passion, and the intimate pillow talk when the body tension has fled many find to be the best part of making love. If being vocal during sex does not come naturally, it can be learned. When it's done to please a lover, the payback is considerable!

For me it's more pleasurable if she is vocal, even during foreplay. I like to know that what I am doing is what she likes. It doesn't require a monologue or screaming. Nothing fake. Just something to let me know I am not way out in left field or if I am that I need to zero in on home.

———

Try this: Both of you are blindfolded, naked, on the bed. No touching. Think about sex. Describe what you see in your mind's eye. Removing the visual prompts forces you to rely on words to communicate. It won't be as embarrassing as talking face to face, and as you get more and more excited you'll get more and more expressive.

———

I love it when my lover talks to me during the act. I had one lover who told me how beautiful I was during the whole thing and I have never felt more loved. If you want your lover to do more of it, why don't you suggest reading erotic stories out loud to one another to get the hang of it? Maybe she'll get the hint. Even if she doesn't it makes for great foreplay. Try *eroticstories.com.*

———

It isn't necessary to use "dirty" words. One's language can be passionate and quite chaste with the use of flowery terms and imagery or just the tone of voice. Another very good thing about making talk sexy is that it makes it easy to ask for specific things without sounding clinical or demanding. If a woman asks a lover to "stroke my clitoris softly with that velvety tongue of yours. Oh yeah! just like *that!*" the receiver of those words will probably consider it a favor done for him or her.

———

I am so fortunate. I have a wife who helps me maximize her pleasure by telling me the effect of every nuance of my lovemaking. She is not afraid to say, "That's too hard" or, "A little farther up" or, "Not so fast." But it takes a confident woman to tell her man what feels good at that moment.

———

My pillow pal is unlike any of my previous partners: He doesn't put me on a pedestal, he doesn't treat me like a fragile piece of crystal, and he talks to me in a decidedly ungentlemanly manner when we're in bed. (He treats me with respect outside the bedroom.) And let me tell you, I absolutely love it. No one else has ever called me a dirty little slut before, and it drives me crazy in a very good way. The weird thing is, I actually act like a "slut" when I'm with him—I'm way more uninhibited than with guys who merely say I'm lovely and do the cozy, warm, not very scorching lovemaking routine.

———

Sometimes two talkers will be attracted to one another, but rarely. I love to talk during sex, but my wife doesn't so I've mostly stopped. I'll fantasize things she might say to me if I want to come quickly. She has made some effort. Just a few hours ago, before I left for a business conference, she pulled my pants down and pushed me to the bed and climbed on top of me. When I was getting ready to come I told her so, and she whispered, "Yes, come inside me now." Every now and then if she's really coming hard during penetration she'll cry out, "Do me!" That was cool. My ideal lover would be someone who was a real screamer and very verbal and loved to talk nasty nonstop. In my dreams....

———

I would love to hear more talking in my sex life. Sometimes seems like I am the only one there.

Sex Toys

We have made a giant stride forward in that dildos and vibrators and such are now called "sex toys," suggesting fun and games, and are no longer referred to as "marital aides," which brings to mind a medical appliance, like a truss, that is unavailable to the uncoupled. Another major advancement is that shopping for sex toys, instead of requiring furtive trips to the seedy side of town, can now be done in smartly designed romantic boutiques or online in complete privacy. There is absolutely no surer way for a pre-orgasmic woman to reach her goal than with a "personal massager." Toys are not for everyone's sensibilities, but keep an open mind. You didn't always know how to use a yo-yo either.

There is no guesswork with a vibrator, just turn it on and *Wow!* Yank every last ounce of satisfaction out of an orgasm. I 'd be interested to know why any woman would make a conscious decision not to use one. That kinda like saying I would take a whiff of a steak but not eat it rare . . . or, take a shower but not use soap, or go watch a sunset but wear dark glasses. You just miss the most that can be gotten out of it.

———

The softer "jelly-type" vibrators feel gorgeous, but they are difficult to keep clean, no matter how well you wash them. If you are prone to vaginitis or yeast infections, you might want to consider a harder plastic vibrator. They are easier to clean and are more hygienic in general.

———

I have two. One vibrates harder and the other one produces a finer, more buzzy-like feeling. I like the buzzy one better. I would have never been able to make that choice without actually using the product, so you may purchase something that doesn't *do* it for you. You may have to try a couple of different ones.

———

Have some fun buying toys. Throw caution to the wind. Give the person at the counter something to smile about. I'm sure they've seen stranger things. Look where they work!

———

As for vibrators, if you simply seek external stimulation, the wand types seem very popular. They tend to be a bit noisy. The cordless ones seem a lot more convenient. If you wish to experiment with penetration, I suggest one of the soft latex types shaped like a phallus, definitely a multi-speed as this offers the most versatility. This type offers a person external stimulation with options. Some folks are sensitive to latex products, so be aware if this is a problem. There are others constructed of soft materials, but they are not as pliable. There is also another type that can be worn under your clothing and offers hands-free external stimulation. They are virtually noise-free, and the intensity can be adjusted to your desire. I have seen them advertised as Butterflies.

———

I know the latest generation of dildos has a variety of futuristic not-phallus like shapes—ranging from dolphins (some even squirting!) to strange-looking shapes I wouldn't know how to define! I think some you can even put on your mantelpiece and no one would even know it was a dildo!

CHAPTER 7

Intercourse

I almost titled this chapter "The Main Event," but I don't want to add to the popular misconception that penis into vagina (and out of and into again) is what sex is all about—that, in fact, sex equals intercourse, and all the other good stuff is just so much parsley on the meat-and-potatoes plate of human sexuality. Actually, in sifting through letters and online posts while putting this book together, I found that there really wasn't a significant amount of discussion about the act of heterosexual intercourse itself beyond the relative merits of this or that position and when, in the scheme of a relationship, it's best to happen. We touched upon this in the initial chapters.

I want to add an anecdote here that has stayed with me all my years as a sex educator. When I first started volunteering on the phone lines for San Francisco Sex Information, almost twenty-five years ago, I overheard a middle-aged man describing the act to a youngster thus: "The vagina slowly envelops the penis and brings it into itself." Puts a whole new perspective on intercourse, doesn't it?

The Old In and Out

It's amazing, given the fact that most people equate intercourse with sex itself, the birds-and-bees mystery of where babies come from, and that thing "everyone else's parents did except mine," that more people haven't written about it to my column or at the online Forum. Intercourse, once it has a place in an adult's life, seems to assume less importance. Perhaps it's like the quality of air one breathes—of no importance unless you're not getting any. Then it becomes crucial!

The missionary position remains one of the best means of holding, hugging, and being close to your partner. All the other ruffles and flourishes are great, but there's just something wonderful about connecting face to face. I think it's that connection—the close face-to-face aspect—that makes missionary position sex the most intimate. Sometimes I suspect people engage in more exotic behaviors as a means to avoid that intimacy. It's the eye contact, moaning in your partner's ear, whispering "I love you" that makes this position so wonderful. This is the way for partners to really emotionally connect, not just physically couple.

———

I don't get much real juice out of being inert under a man's body; I never have. I like moving, and it is all the better when varied with the more gentle closeness as I bend down for kisses. He says he likes being able to lie back and just suck up all the sensations and attention when I'm on top.

———

A pillow under the hips can bring a smile to your lips.

———

Most girls I know just don't prefer

The boys who act like power drills;

Though hard and fast sure can be nice

It's *tenderness* that gives them thrills.

If you're too slow or gentle, you can always get more firm or force-ful, but if you're too firm or forceful, going back to slow or gentle often doesn't work. In other words, if you start out with high-speed pound-ing, and one partner wants slow and sensuous motions, then it's very difficult to slow down—sensitivity has already been lost.

———

The virtues of switching back and forth between penetration and cunnilingus are often underrated. If I've come earlier than I intended, or if my partner hasn't been able to come from penetration, I'm more than happy to go down on her immediately after orgasm. I think that men can get over their distaste for going down on someone inside of whom they've just ejaculated. (Of course, if condoms with nonoxynol-9 were used, it's a different story.)

———

If you've never had unprotected sex, you should know that a lot of things will change when you stop using condoms. Many positions that didn't do much for me when I was using protection, like woman-on-top, are far more rewarding without a condom. There's not much that *isn't* better without a condom (though my orgasms were sometimes more intense with one), but it's surprising how much better some positions become.

———

I don't think most men are bothered too much, or turned off, by the sound of air noisily escaping a woman's vagina. However, I had a partner who would laugh for nearly a full minute whenever it hap-pened, and that withered my erection almost without fail!

———

Don't underestimate the extent to which the fear of pregnancy can dampen your enjoyment. I used to suffer from severe postcoital despair until my partner went on the pill; I didn't really realize how afraid I had been of getting her pregnant.

———

It's always a shame to encounter a well-endowed guy who seems to think his extra inches entitle him to just *coast* on his length. I want to whip out a user's manual (would that there were such a thing!) and show him that, by god, there *is* more than one "setting" for that "power tool" he's so obviously infatuated with.

———

Variety and surprise are marvelous, effective elements—the ability to mix up speed, depth of penetration, and approach (rough versus tender).

———

Eyes closed, I like to begin with him going in, very, very slowly, then back out again, very, very slowly, feeling every single inch enter me. At first feeling the tip touch my lips, then with a little pressure, the head slowly slides in, spreading me apart; then the rim slips in … *slowwwwwly* pulls out again, then back in, ahh, now the shaft makes its way in, gentle, slow, and soft so I can squeeze and create the perfect visual of the shape, size, and texture!

———

If anyone has ever found "doggie-style" to be a big turn-on in theory, but a little too detached (no eye contact, no getting to see his or her face) in reality, try it in front of a mirror. It makes a big difference. Works nicely for anal sex too.

———

Having sexual timing problems? Can't climax during intercourse? May I suggest a technique described in Laura Haydon's book entitled something like *How to Please a Woman Every Time (and Make Her Beg for More)*? OK, cheesy title, but Ms. Haydon claims that this technique works for every woman who has been unable to climax during intercourse. It may also help with early ejaculation problems. If it doesn't work, it's still a helluva lot of fun! He inserts the head of his cock, just barely. (I recommend the missionary position for this, for the eye contact.) He slides the head in and almost out with a not-too-fast and not-too-slow speed. Keep the action steady for several minutes; then he should insert his cock a half-inch to an inch further in, and continue the steady in-out movement (but not all the way out-keep the strokes short and concentrated on one small section of your vagina, and he should remember to angle himself toward your frontal "wall"). After a few more minutes, he should go in a *leeeeetle* bit further, continue the short, steady in-outs, then a few minutes later, a little further, and so on and so on. Somewhere along the way, if Haydon's claim is true, you should find yourself having your first mind-blowing orgasm of your (literally) fucking life. For the record, I tried this on my S.O. once (she was already orgasmic during intercourse, but I didn't hold that against her). After about thirty minutes, when I was almost completely inside her (like I suggested, take your time!), I thought it was a very pleasant failure—she was enjoying herself (as was I), but there was no sign of the tension that she was building toward the big O. All of a sudden, her eyes got wide and she was screaming like a banshee! After her orgasm semi-subsided, she managed to mutter, "I have never . . . in my life . . ." and let the sentence trail off from there.

———

There are a couple of positions that can help you get that "fuller" feel. My wife and I both enjoy me being on top, with her squeezing her legs together and my legs on the outside of hers. I end up almost sitting on top in that position, and it's very comfortable for both (we discovered this position when she was pregnant), because there is no pressure put on her above her waist. All my weight is on her legs and some on my hands and arms. Recently we discovered this can work with her on her stomach as well and actually provides deeper penetration than if I'm just trying to lie on top of her from behind.

———

I prefer my orgasm to come when she is on top, squatting with an up-and-down motion. I love the stimulation along the entire shaft from head to balls, and I can also control the motion with my own movement.

———

Me and hubby were making love last night and found a new position that we love! He was lying catty-corner on the bed on his side, and I was lying the opposite way on my back, like we were making the letter X. I had one leg between his legs and the other thrown over his hip. It was a great position because we could both touch each other and stimulate other areas of our bodies and we could both move easily. I loved it!

———

The only way (other than oral or manual or by vibrator) my partner can orgasm with intercourse is when she sits on top and hits her G-Spot with backward pressure. Hard for me to hold on without orgasming myself before she reaches hers, but now I can outlast her any day. I learned to be multi-orgasmic and found a premature ejaculation cure at *www.OrgasmControl.com.*

———

I've had very intimate woman-to-woman sex with my partner in the top and bottom positions. The woman on top usually moves around a bit to find the best spot, while opening her partner's labia and pressing herself clit to clit. It's hard to stay in position sometimes, and we end up in the side-to-side position. It's very sensual.

———

Scissors position, vulva to vulva! Hands clutching each other's hands, pulling each other closer. Both my partner and I have hairless pubes, so things can get pretty slickery. Add some warm lube.

———

Lie on your sides, facing each other. (You can roll around as much as you like, but this will help me explain it.) Put one of your thighs between her legs and let her do the same. This way, you can both push against each others' thighs in whatever way feels good to you, and you can feel each other on you (heat, moisture, pressure—depending on how much fabric is in the way). It's very mutual, very close (no hard appendages coming between you). You can experiment with it all you like, but in the end, this is the nicest thing to me. It allows for a level of comfort that you can't get with oral sex, because you can kiss, hug, and be completely against each other while getting off. Life is good. Enjoy!

———

One little trick I have discovered in lovemaking is what I call "the wiggle." It's accomplished by lying flat, legs stretched straight out. As I alternate between extending one leg as far as possible, then the other, my erect penis goes back and forth sideways as my pelvis rotates. My wife has always had three or four orgasms, but "the wiggle" has increased their intensity.

———

I lie on my left side facing my S.O., and she is 90 degrees from me on her back. Her right leg goes over my right hip, and my left leg goes under her left leg. I penetrate her while I stimulate her clit with my right hand. Now I vary the speed and intensity of the thrust depending on how crazy she goes. Sometimes I go real slow and do circles on her clit. I know it's done right when she grabs a pillow to muffle her screams. Then I have to replace the pillows, because she bites holes in them.

———

I lie on my back, my legs spread and her on top, facing me with her legs together (kind of a reverse missionary). After enjoying this for a few minutes I bend my knees to about 45 degrees and lift my feet about a foot off the bed, resulting in my abdominals tensing. *Immediately* when I do this the sensations increase, and I'll climax within 120 seconds. They seem to be more intense climaxes as well. One of the nice things about this position is fantasizing about role reversal: I fantasize that I'm being penetrated. I'm not sure what does it for me, the fantasizing, the tightening of the abdominals, the position itself, but it really has been amazing.

———

Doggie-style, like anal sex, should be controlled by your partner. Position yourself, with slight insertion, and then let her do the pumping. You feel like you are getting an ass blow job, while she controls her own climax, which is usually superb.

———

I had an ex who was more than a foot taller than me. Just meant my ass and hips had to be pushed up higher in the air if we wanted to do rear entry without pain. Try some different angles. Sometimes it isn't penetration and depth that feels best (or so he said), but the different pressures on different areas of his shaft and head.

———

I find that if I lean forward with my head to the side on a pillow, and my bottom in the air, I can come. It allows for deeper penetration. The more I arch my back and put my butt in the air, the better it feels. That may have something to do with being wide open for the taking.

———

If you feel comfortable with doggie-style, it frees your hands and arms so that you can rub your clit. It's a fail-proof method for me!

———

I can't seem to finger myself during doggie without falling on my face and losing all sense of rhythm, so I gave up and found another trick. If he'll give you some control over the angle of his thrusting, pull in your tummy, curve your back and butt, and then rub your clit and G-spot down the underside of his cock when you meet his thrusts, instead of meeting them straight on. You'll get a lot more stimulation this way. It's so easy to do, you won't even break the rhythm. Some men like to control the angle, so if he fusses about what you're doing to his system don't be shy. Tell him you're making it easier for him to make you come! And especially tell him how good it feels that way (if you like it), and you'll be able to show him the difference it makes in no time at all! My hubby is very strict about controlling everything about our sex life and has a preferred angle, but I still manage to throw him a few curves sometimes! Even if I don't get the chance to do it long enough to come, it makes doing doggie so much better!

———

For sex, anything over and above clean sheets and clean bodies is just gilt and is unnecessary!

Sexual Housekeeping

With condom use more prevalent, and female ejaculation gaining notoriety, fairly soon blame for the wet spot will be shifted from him entirely to her. Usually, however, it is a product of joint effort . . . so to speak.

Keep a stack of towels nearby and when you're finished making love, wipe yourselves up, then reach over and drop that puppy on the floor. That's right. On the floor. You can do that now. Mom's not around anymore to lecture you on keeping your room clean. You can take the used towel to the hamper in the morning after a night of restful sleep.

———

At the very least I get up and get her a warm washcloth and a towel. If she needs to go to the bathroom, well, there's just nothing that I can help her with there.

———

Most of the time we keep a towel nearby, and she asks me to pull out and come on her stomach. That way she doesn't have to deal with the dreaded drip. Works for me too, because I stay clean and I kind of enjoy coming on her rather than in her.

———

In England, it's part of the post-sex ritual for many guys that they clean everything up for the lady, using tissue in the operational areas.

Seems to be an accepted thing that it's his responsibility. Kind of a nice, loving touch, I think.

———

What about having some diaper wipes, or something similar, plus a towel by the bed? That's my simplistic solution. You'll have to take care of the wipes and towel later, but the immediate problem is solved.

———

A friend once said that "towels are for married people, sheets-only are for lovers." I remember an old song from when I was a teenager called "My Boyfriend's Back." That pretty quickly got turned into "My boyfriend's back and there's gonna be laundry."

CHAPTER 8

Oral Sex on a Woman

One of the most amazing discoveries many women make is that there are men who go way beyond being willing to provide oral sex in the name of being a good lover, but who actually love the act itself and seek it out for their own pleasure as well as their partners'. Isn't it delightful that Nature provided willing givers as well as willing receivers ... and isn't it lucky for everyone when a couple is made up of one of each!

Pleasuring the woman is important, and is I guess the main thing, but I have to say the best thing about it for me is coming into such intimate contact with pure femaleness. It's hard to imagine anything more intensely female than that part of a woman, especially when the rest of her is enjoying it so much. And being doused with that aroma, which I hate to wash off, is arousing and satisfying in a deeply natural sort of way.

———

Phagophobists (those who have fear of eating) are often afraid because they don't know how to enjoy it. People have fears about giving a woman oral sex because society glamorizes only the visual and tangible aspects of the vagina, while insulting its tastes and scents. No anthropomorphic imagery—not a rose, not a scallop, not a peach—properly honors the goddess we call pussy. It is a living, changing microcosm of the woman's soul. As she ascends to a state of pure sexuality, her pheromones overpower everything. The taste gets better, the smell gets better, and the sex gets better. Arousal comes a lot quicker with a genuine sense of commitment.

———

Start high, lots of gentle kissing on her face and neck and ears and shoulders. Lots of gently feeling her skin all over. Work your way down to her breasts and back and tummy, kissing and feeling and touching, and go slowly. Work your way around, down her thighs and back up. Kiss and massage her feet (no tickling). Work your way back up her legs, kissing and feeling and touching. Get closer. Go slow. Back off down her thighs and knees. Start back up, kissing and feeling and touching. Kiss her lips, and whatever you do, don't act like you're starved to death. Kiss her womanhood. Alternate gentle kissing and sucking with quick flicks of your tongue. Constantly think soft, warm, gentle, loving, intimate, tender thoughts toward your beloved. It is what you are trying to communicate. Make sure you vary your loving actions. Don't just lie there and flick away. Be imaginative and explore her whole body, discover new ways of kissing, touching, feeling, but always return to her womanhood. Spend most of your time there, but make sure you adore her whole body. After the explosions of love, be sure to hold her for a long time. Adore her body. This follow-up is critical. It seals your and her loving emotions and sets the tone for the next time.

―――

If a sore neck is cramping your style, a change in position might help. You could try having her sit in a chair or on a barstool, and then crouch between her legs. A similar position can be taken if she scooches her bottom to the edge of the bed and you crouch on the floor. You can try to approach her from the side, over her thigh and hip. In this position your neck won't be at such an uncomfortable angle. If your tongue is getting tired, you might be making it work too hard. Try kissing her clitoris like you would kiss her mouth, tenderly. Experiment by flicking against her clit with the pointed tip of your tongue, then a softened tip; snuggle your tongue gently against the length of her clit. Purse your lips and *gently* suck the nub into your mouth, again and again. Use your tongue and lips to sensually explore the ridge and sides of the clitoral hood. Place a trail of wet kisses down either side of her labia, interspersed by a lick here, a suck there, a gentle nip. Don't feel it's necessary to "drill" her vagina nonstop with your tongue. Your fingers can do the same thing, leaving your mouth free to explore the other delights of her nethers. Mix your techniques up according to her response. Some women do not respond well to direct stimulation on the exposed glans of the clitoris (the pearly nub of tissue below the hood). If she's one of them, she may prefer more attention to the hood. Experiment and find out what works.

―――

Don't just paint the fence, practice writing the alphabet. No matter what position you find yourself in!

―――

If oral stimulation gets her to orgasm, then by all means go for it. However, do consider that if you penetrate her as she is orgasming, the subsequent orgasm will *really* rock her world.

―――

The best way to do cunnilingus from the top during 69 is to use the tip of your tongue on the area just below the clitoris, letting your lower lip just graze the tip of her clit. Also, use a finger gently inserted just as far as the first knuckle in her entrance. Move it gently in and out and around. At this point she usually forgets to suck, but who cares?

———

Cunnilingus from the top, as one might suspect, is a whole different animal. The map, after all, is upside down. Imagine Lewis and Clark searching for the Southeast Passage! Nevertheless, the assiduous male student of Oral Arts may find the journey less arduous if his ardor includes the following:

1. *Hands.* The backs of a woman's thighs, knees, and calves, as well as her buttocks, all long neglected during traditional woman-on-back cunnilingus, are now treasure troves for soft gliding fingertips. Whatever's going on orally, tease and tickle the swell of her calf, the nook of her knee, the strong, surprisingly ticklish hamstring.

2. *Labia—part two.* Er, that's a pun. Anyway. I favor an all-over-the-place approach to vulva-licking in this position. Kiss and lick up and down one vaginal lip, then the other, then slide the tongue into her vagina, but instead of licking backward toward the G-spot, lick down into the tailbone. Let your chin gently rub against the hood of her clitoris, just to let her know you aren't lost in Missouri (see reference to Southeast Passage, supra), and you're going to get to the promised land.

3. When it's finally time to get to the clit, things really get topsy-turvy. So we'll just fight top with turve, and let our tongue become our upper lip, and versa vice. Slide the tongue downward from the base of the clit to the tip, then flick outward. Slide it down the left side, and flick likewise. Slide down the right et cetera. The true *cunnus* aficionado, whether he's experienced it once or 10,000 times, will find that the hardness and

length of the clitoris in the aroused state is a delightful surprise. While all that sliding is going on, let's stop with the fingertip-gliding and grab the lady's butt cheeks firmly in the palms of our hands. After all, every act of oral sex has elements of surrender and power, and we're often not sure who's the surrenderer and who's the surrenderee. Nevertheless, if your tongue is doing what it ought to be doing, she's going to be as restless as a willow in a windstorm, so take charge, take heart, hell, take the A train, but take her ass in your hands like you mean it. (Yes, the surrenderer-surrenderee thing becomes problematic during 69, which is why that position is not for the squeamish.) While the tongue is doing that sliding thing, the upper lip should be dancing a gavotte on the tip of the clit and hood, which should, in turn, produce hip-bucking action on the part of milady (finger insertion at this point is optional but frequently desirable). Synchronize the tongue sliding and the lip gavotting until she's in a frenzy, then don't stop.

———

Before getting to the clit, I like sucking up the labia into my mouth and running my tongue between the lips. Then suck up one lip at a time. There's the perineum not to be forgotten. Finally I like to lick the clitoral hood. I think it's effective to make sucking noises while performing this. I get hard just thinking about it.

———

Recently my girlfriend and I had finished a rather intense episode of lovemaking. She was standing naked in a full-length mirror, combing her hair. The shape of her body and her ass turned me on, so I walked behind her and began a slow trail of kisses down her back, waist, and ass. When I got to her ass she turned around and guided my head between her legs. She stood over me as I kneeled and ate her out. Her orgasm was so powerful I wondered if might be safer if we moved away from the mirror.

———

Start out slowly. Kiss and taste your way from her belly to the pubic mound. Women are very sensitive around the whole area, and most love a little teasing. Try this and explore for a while and become adjusted to her smell. If this doesn't work, try some edible massage oil rubbed over her first. Can be great fun just by itself. Don't put too much pressure on yourself or feel bad if it doesn't work out the first few times.

I prefer to be lying on my back because I tend to have very intense orgasms during oral, and I like to be able to enjoy the experience without worrying about falling down. For some reason, finger penetration isn't a big deal for me. The tongue action on my inner lips and clit is enough. In fact, fingers almost distract from the focus of the tongue. I also like to have my lips massaged firmly and sucked. One great technique is to suck the clit between pursed lips and flick it with the tongue—that pushes me over the edge!

I love to be on my back at the edge of the bed with my lover on the floor between my spread legs. I love to be licked as well as fingered . . . my lips spread and played with . . . my tunnel explored . . . my clit licked and pulled at with soft lips . . . *mmmmmmmm.*

If my husband has his nose buried between my thighs, I don't want to think he's doing it because he *has* to, but because he *wants* to. Telling me that I look, smell, and taste good is just one way of verifying that for me—provided it's said with all sincerity. In addition, this removes the burden of wondering if I smell bad down there. With that troublesome thought out of the way, I can relax and sink into the pleasure of our lovemaking. It's a two-way street of course. My husband's testes smell like a rich, red wine, and I think it's an intoxicatingly sexy aroma.

I have never tasted a woman who was sweet, except when I used some types of "fun" stuff. That can make things more exciting, but a woman usually tastes a little salty, and as she gets even more excited, well, it's hard to describe the flavor. The more important thing for me is that my wife has incredible orgasms, multiples as well, and that excites me like crazy, so I love giving her head! That is the main key: you've got to love it. If she thinks for just a moment that this is a chore, she will not be able to get that out of her mind and it will blow the whole experience. If you really want to love the taste, find some of those edible creams on the Internet or your local sex shoppe.

I enjoy giving oral sex to a woman more than anything else now, but I remember the first time I did it. I asked to try it and she said OK. She held open her lips and I kissed her right on the clit. I remember her moaning instantly; my reaction was that it didn't really taste like anything but it was sticky. It kinda turned me off. Remembering the very pronounced moan, I tried again and just used the tip of my tongue. That went OK and she had an extremely intense orgasm. I gradually progressed, so that now when I eat a woman I get my whole face in there, tongue inside her as far as I can (that's a stronger taste), and when I'm done I have pussy juice all over my face from my nose to my chin, and it's *fabulous!*

I once had a great orgasm while giving my wife oral sex. The whole experience—taste, feel, smell—was a great turn-on.

The kisses men give are a direct sign of what they are like when they give oral sex. It seems the more passionate, snake-like, and exploring he is with his tongue when he kisses me, the more likely he will be to do the same when he goes down.

Many women love to be teased. So, when you get to the Holy Gates, hold off on the main event. Nestle your nose in her bush, assuming she has one. Make yummy noises—let her know that her smell excites you. Delicately caress the bottom of her vagina with your tongue. Slide your nose in past the fur, and caress her lips with it. Take one labium (she'll love your Latin) between your lips, and rest your tongue on the ridge. Slide up and down, up and down. Change to the other side, and repeat. Then make an O with your lips, and invite your tongue into her inner sanctum. Swirl your tongue around, in, out—gently, gently—until she's all wet and so are you. Raise your head, lifting your tongue up and out, with a teasing flick at her clit, then go back to her pussy. Again. Once more, with feeling. That's it, keep it up. When she starts pulling your hair out, it's time to concentrate on the clit. Use your lips to gently push back her hood and labia, and butterfly that love button with your tongue. Cock your head left and right, so you're always hitting a different spot. (Always take more time with everything than you think you should, by the way—hey, you're not going anywhere, right?) Using your lower lip to cover your teeth, let your jaw brace against her pubic bone. At the same time, use your upper lip to push back her hood. Keep butterflying, but with a little more pressure. Keep cocking your head, but a little faster, and make the angles shallower, until you're straight up practically all the time. Use your upper lip to press against her hood, stroking it up and down. Your butterfly should now be stinging like a very insistent bee, but a honeybee, nevertheless. Somewhere along the way, nirvana should be reached (we hope!). After she's come, don't forget to lavish her vulva with kisses for being so incredibly wonderful.

———

I have to say I like a finger inside, or just holding on to my legs for dear life.

———

I love it when he explores every orifice lovingly, wantonly, hungrily. Alternating with his fingers deep inside me while his mouth is on my clit and then his fingers rubbing my clit while his tongue is deep inside me. Just as long as he's enjoying himself and showing it, while I'm enjoying whatever he is doing to me and letting him know it, his hands can roam all over my body.

———

First start out slowly with what most people call foreplay. Once your head is between her legs, spread the outer lips and gently kiss her all over. Insert your tongue into her vagina and savor the flavor of her body. Work your way upward and start licking her clitoris, gently, gentlemen, gently. This is a highly sensitive spot. (It is best if you continue to lick at her clitoris at all times.) As you feel her sexual craving grow again gently massage the opening of her vagina with your fingers. As her vagina becomes lubricated insert your forefinger into her vagina about an inch and a half; point the tip of your finger upward and gently massage the upper vaginal wall. Once she is in the sexual hot zone, remove your finger from her vagina and place it on her anus. Insert your finger into her anus one or two inches, and place the tip of your finger onto the wall that separates the anus and vaginal cavities. Pulling your finger in and out, rub this wall vigorously so as to make contact with the upper vaginal wall. If done properly this will drive her into a sexual frenzy, but you are not done yet. *Remember at all times you are lashing at her engorged clitoris.* Finally the *coup de grâce*, while performing all of the above with your other hand, reach up and take the nipple of her breast and roll it between your thumb and forefinger. She will have an orgasm with no equal.

———

Start out gently; this is performed for her pleasure. Don't worry about yourself. Think only of her. Her pleasure is your pleasure.

———

I enjoy going down on my wife, and if she never went down on me, she'd still have to pry my head from between her legs at times.

———

What is it that makes us want to perform it on others? Is it just the sensation of something swelling on our tongue, the slight taste of salt, the feeling of our nose on that cushion of hair? Or, is it the reaction we get from our partner—the thrashing and the moaning that lets us know she really, really likes what we are doing, the ego rush of having someone call your name until 2 A.M.? What is it that makes us say with a knowing wink, "Moving your mouth on someone until your jaw goes numb ain't really a *bad* thing..."?

CHAPTER 9

Oral Sex on a Man

I t's pretty obvious that blow jobs are not about puffing and are not necessarily work, and that something or someone who sucks is not necessarily a bad thing at all. So much for slang as communication. Once upon a time the issue was whether or not to indulge in oral sex. While for many it still is, increasingly it's not whether or when to but how. As always with sex, what constitutes a satisfying experience is highly personal, and the owner of the genitals on which attention is being lavished is always the ultimate authority. Even if you've never before heard of the practice of genital kissing, you will be an expert on the matter when you finish reading the following comments.

Don't think of it as a blow job. When you think "blow job" it implies "dirty" to some. Also, the term makes you think in mechanical terms, not loving terms. And it shouldn't be a job. The man's penis is just another part of his body. It really isn't any different from any other body part. It has special functions like all the parts do. (An old engineering joke has it that a civil engineer designed the penis. Who else but a civil engineer would combine waste removal and recreational facilities through a single pipeline?) Anyway, the penis and groin area are all very sensitive to touch. Especially a woman's touch. I wonder if women really know how powerful their touch is to a man's groin area, balls, and penis? Or how loving it can feel to a man? Start touching along the inner thighs and *lightly* stroking the balls. All kinds of motion, circular strokes, by the way, fingers first here. Then use your tongue and lips to stroke and kiss him. You don't have to swallow the whole thing, or anything else. If you're worried about cleanliness, don't be afraid to wash him. Just do it in a loving manner. This can be very enjoyable to a guy. Think of giving your affection and care and love for him through his manhood. You're giving something of worth and value and intimacy to him.

———

The very first few times I got a blow job I couldn't come from it. Finally one girlfriend combined a hand job with it and I did. Then as I got more I learned that if I would relax and focus on enjoying it (and I like to watch her mouth move up and down my dick), it really is fantastic. It's much more subtle a sensation than any other form of stimulation, and it still takes me longer to come from a BJ than from anything else.

———

I don't mind when my husband does it as long as I have a hand on his penis so that it doesn't gag me. I hold it in one hand to control how far I take it in.

———

What seems to work with my partner is (1) Choose your moment. A quick blow job has its place, but a long one is twice as nice. (2)

Choose your style. Sometimes it's appropriate to dive right to the heart of the matter. Other times, it's far more enjoyable to take the long way 'round the bed. (3) Choose your position. My personal favorite is to have him lie at the edge of the bed while I kneel between his legs. This allows me plenty of space to move around and gives me clear access to all my favorite parts. Sometimes it's nice to try something different, just for a change of pace. Your partner can stand, sit, kneel, lie. Whatever position he chooses, make sure it's one you'll be comfortable in as well. It's hard to give a good blow job when you've got a crick in your neck. When it's time to begin, don't go right for his cock. Increase his excitement and anticipation by teasing him for as long as you can both stand it. Lightly tickle his thighs, scrotum, and perineum with your hands. Rub your hair over his body, trap his cock in it, brush it over his balls. Use your voice to excite him even more—tell him how much you're looking forward to this mutual pleasure. Blow hot air over his sac and the head of his cock. Suck the air in from around his cock (note the slight flavor). Bury your nose in his sac and inhale deeply. Let him know via your actions that you love what you're doing. Your mouth, lips, tongue, and teeth (if he likes that) can be used in a number of ways to provide different sensations. Use your hands as well to stroke his shaft, and cup and massage his testes as you suck, lick, flutter, diddle, kiss, and nibble. The primary place of attention should be on the underside of his cock, right beneath the head. Try sucking the flesh there into your mouth and flutter it with your tongue. Intersperse this with deep thrusts, then lollipop licks against the head. Lightly (!) graze your teeth against his crown. Enjoy, have fun, take your time. If he's open to the experience, you can also incorporate anal play into your actions. Press the flat of your tongue against his anus; flutter the silky skin there with your tongue. Come back up and devour the length of his shaft before returning to your rimming efforts. If he's enjoying himself, you can insert a finger or toy into his anus. Use a lubricant and go slowly if this is a new experience for both of you. The prostate can also be stimulated via the perineum. Use your fingers to press in a pulsing motion there. Use your fingertips to explore the base of his penis. Pay close attention to his response, that spoken and that conveyed through body language. Adjust your actions accordingly. Keep playing—here, there, and everywhere—until he cries "Uncle!"

———

There are times that I want my man to talk to dirty to me—I mean call me his bitch and he is my pimp, and at that time I want him to somewhat force his penis in my mouth. *But* there are times that I want it to be my game . . . if you know what I mean!

———

I don't mind it if a lover suggests to me by his actions that he wants me to go down on him. I just don't like having my head pushed. I love falling down to my knees (Is that submissive, or what?) and grabbing his member with my mouth, all on my own. I've got a small mouth and I compensate very well with my hands.

———

I had a sex buddy (for lack of a better term) in college who introduced me to the wonderful world of blow jobs done with a cough drop in the woman's mouth. She said she read about it and wanted to try it, and who am I to say no?

———

Don't try to swallow the entire thing. Imagine that you love his penis and treat it that way. Play with his balls and stroke him at the same time. Lastly, don't try to make him come. Use it only as foreplay leading up to the grand entrance.

———

I really enjoy giving head, whether as a prelude to other things or the whole enchilada, so to speak. If the taste of his cock is a turn-off for you—wash it. Have that be part of the act, and if he gets offended, don't go down. A clean partner is rule number 1 for most people in enjoying oral sex. If he's clean enough but you still want a flavor additive—I'd suggest Nutella (it's my favorite for this sort of thing). A little bit goes a long way, it's not too sweet, it's not suck-able—so your jaw will get a rest. Gloss a little bit (use it sparingly) over his cock and balls and you'll be licking for a long time. And the licking part is nice for them. If your jaw hurts, that could mean your mouth is small or it could be an indication that he takes a very long time. When my partner takes a *really* long time I'll start to get a jaw ache too. At that point I usually pull off a little bit and start licking away. He doesn't mind.

The first blow job I ever had was her first too, and she just wasn't ready to take the whole thing in, so she kind of sucked the front of it. My goodness, it was nice. There are very few ways you can go wrong with a cock if you're using something warm, soft, and wet.

Enthusiasm is a must. Ladies, please don't act as though you are doing us a favor when you give us a BJ. We want to feel as though you want to do it, you love doing it.

Of course, even the best technique can't make up for lack of enthusiasm. If you love what you're doing, let him know. Many men find eye-contact to be exciting, as well as masturbating him against various parts of your own body: thighs, breasts, clit, labia, lips. You might also want to try a cock ring, or tickling him with a feather, or masturbating him with a silk handkerchief. In fact, there's no reason why you can't incorporate a number of these sorts of activities into your fellating moments.

Men are very visual creatures. Let us watch. Have the lights on, have your hair held back or to the side—don't let your hair act as a curtain.

The use of your hand is important too. It should be involved in the action. Use one hand to stroke his shaft and the other, if you get the balance right, to play with his balls. (It's quite possible that a blow job is a new sensation to him and the pressure is not the same as manual stimulation. So, work on the manual part at the same time if you can.)

————

Deep throating is nice but it isn't necessary for a good blow job. And swallowing is a must for some, no big deal for others, and a complete turn-off for some. Do what *you* like and what *you're* comfortable with.

————

I'm not a woman who's comfortable with swallowing (it triggers my gag reflex every time), but I have no objection to him coming in my mouth. As I suck him back to a flaccid state, I simply use my tongue to push the semen out of my mouth—a nearby hand towel takes care of the rest.

————

As he's approaching orgasm, I try to apply a slight upward firm pressure to his perineum, just behind and a bit below the testes—this stimulates the prostate and provides a stronger and longer lasting orgasm.

————

Try gently taking one ball at a time in your mouth, taking your tongue and searching the area, feeling the skin between your lips tightening and growing firmer. Sends hubby through the roof this does; I'm not sure if this is something male-wide or not. But I sure enjoy the soft texture between my lips!

————

I suspect a number of factors could contribute to not climaxing with oral sex. First of all, the sensations may simply be too different from what you're accustomed to. Second, your partner may not be providing you with the specific stimulation you need. Do you feel comfortable asking for what you like? This is the most direct course of action to take. In addition to sucking and licking, she can also incorporate stroking of the shaft and (gentle) stroking of the testes. Some men enjoy stimulation of the perineum—the prostate can also be stimulated through the perineum or more directly through the anus.

One idea that may work well is if your partner can masturbate you almost to climax, and then take you in her mouth. If you are too focused on having an orgasm, that can get in the way. The same thing can happen if your partner is overly concerned with giving you one— sex stops being about pleasure and instead becomes a task to accomplish. If you have any hesitation about "coming in her mouth," it can cause you unconsciously to hold back. For example, if your partner doesn't seem eager to go down on you, this may inhibit you enough that you can't come. I would share your concerns with your partner, and then devote a few nights to some relaxed lovemaking sessions. Rather than working toward a goal of orgasm, simply spend your time slowly pleasuring each other and noting what each of you likes or dislikes. Given a supportive and loving atmosphere, you can learn how to orgasm from head.

———

My wife gives me a BJ almost everyday, sometimes twice a day, and I've got to tell you it is absolutely *G-G-G-R-E-A-T!* I would do anything for her and usually do, but it is so satisfying to start and end the day (sometimes the middle of the day) with a BJ. I know she loves it because she even asks me if I'm ready. And we're in our fifties.

———

Teasing and tantalizing with your tongue is great; however one thing that I have found as I become highly aroused is that I lose a little bit of sensitivity and cannot even feel some of the light licks. So go ahead and lick, but just a little bit firmer. Also, when you suck you can probably suck a little bit more than you realize is comfortable. Just watch the teeth.

———

Saliva, lots of saliva.

———

Running your tongue on the bottom head of the penis while sucking is the quickest way to bring your man to orgasm.

———

If you choose to swallow, which we really do appreciate, continue sucking during orgasm to just after. After that Mister Happy gets a bit too sensitive, or just keep sucking and when it gets too much we will pull away.

———

I enjoy it because of how good it makes the guy feel! To me it's a huge turn-on to see a guy losing control and to ejaculate because of it!

———

What is good about BJs in general? It's nice to be able to just lie back and relax and focus on one's own pleasure for a while. It is also great to not have to restrain oneself from coming too soon.

———

Several things can trigger a gag reflex: deep throat or vigorous thrusting or a hard jet of semen hitting the top of your throat, or simply the taste.

———

Most women can learn to deep throat. It takes time and patience. Mostly it's a matter of learning what triggers your gag reflex and then learning to control it. I taught myself how to deep throat by using a small dildo. It took a couple of weeks to learn the basics.

———

Some of the best blow jobs I've had weren't that deep. You don't have to take that much in to make it amazing. I prefer it as more of a surprise at the end anyway, myself. If you can do it, it can be nice, but it's not the most important aspect. I like it when a woman really has her own style, when you could tell it was her blindfolded. Hey, there's an idea for a fun party game!

———

Just for the heck of it, I thought I would try something different this afternoon while I was playing with my dearly beloved. I moved up next to his side in one of my favorite positions for cock play—him lying on his back, and I with one leg extended beneath his legs and the other curled between our bodies. I began by fondling his testes and penis, and then bent to take him in my mouth. Except I didn't take him in my mouth, instead I captured the tiny fold of skin beneath the head (right where his circumcision scar is), and gently sucked it between my lips while diddling it lightly with my tongue. I then kept that piece of skin in my mouth, sucking gently, butterflying, rolling, and (very) lightly grazing with my teeth as one hand stroked the bottom portion of his shaft and the other rolled and caressed his testes. It took about ten minutes before he had an explosive orgasm. At no time did I follow the pattern of a traditional blow-job—lips over head, move down shaft, pull up, repeat.

Although it's difficult to use coffee because half of it dribbles out, he swore that was the most intense blow job he's received, because of the warmth of my mouth and the liquid warmth of the coffee surrounding him.

Guys love it when you just touch it and talk nasty like, "I bet you like me licking your cock." Just kiss it, stroke it, lick it like candy, all the while talking like an out-of-control slut.

Gentle sucking to extract every last drop of cum from his cock and *gentle* licking of the underside of the head and upper shaft after he's come have always been appreciated by my hubby when I'm finishing up a blow job well done. I love giving him BJs and he knows it! That's a very big turn-on for both of us.

I love to have a woman push the base of my cock that lies just underneath my balls. Most women don't know that the penis begins way back there. I get very hard and tend to ooze pre-cum when this happens. I also love it when a finger is used to rim me or is inserted in me.

Here's a little trick I like sometimes: When he's very close to coming, I like to ease up and use only soft, almost pat-like stimulation with the flat of my tongue against his head. Making a deep, stabbing thrust from time to time as I'm doing so always seems to enhance his pleasure. Sometimes I'll bring him close to the point of orgasm several times, and then ease him back away in this manner. (Enthusiastic sounds and words also seem to be appreciated, as does a position that allows him a clear view of all my adoring ministrations.)

Comes a time in a guy when his dick totally thinks for him, and he may have sworn up and down that he will not come in your mouth, but that involves his being on the verge of coming and then pulling away. Give me a royal break. And if you pull away as he is heaving and squirming, about to explode, isn't that kind of sadistic?

I have had my share of different lovers. I have had the dicks of all of them in my mouth. Although I do not discourage coming in my mouth, and I always swallow, I would love to see the situation where a guy says he will not come in your mouth and then actually keeps that promise. Ha! I say to you. For most of the guys I know, that's half of the fun of a blow job.

My girlfriend has never been able to get me off with a BJ but I *really* enjoy it all the same. I'm not afraid of coming in her mouth, in fact I have masturbated and then she has taken me into her mouth to finish. I just can't come that way.

Oral sex on a man is not necessarily sucking his cock. Lick his balls and inner legs; play with his pubic hair. Hold off on sucking; lick his cock like a lollipop. As you feel him coming, take his cock into your mouth, head only, and then let Nature run its course.

My partner will often pull the skin down my shaft as tightly as she can, and then flick the underside of the shaft with her tongue, and also right at the base of the head. It is almost like having a vibrator placed at the base of my penis. She will take that fold of skin and gently suck on it until I am coming in full glory. It makes for quite a visual and intense orgasm.

I tend to begin by planting wet, open-mouthed kisses on his shaft and over the bulb of his cock. I then switch to an up, up, up licking stroke interspersed with more wet kisses, tongue swirls, taking his head completely into my mouth, and deep intermittent thrusts down his shaft as far as I am comfortable. He helps by not holding my head or thrusting his penis into my mouth.

I really like it when my partner licks the area between the balls and anus. This is great for fantasy too—I can fantasize about what it feels like to be a woman receiving oral sex, my wife can fantasize about giving oral to a woman. It's great for building sexual energy to a much higher level before stimulating the cock to orgasm.

If I care about a guy, specifically about his pleasure, he's a candidate for a blow job. And I'm psyched about it almost always. The only time I'm not interested is if he shows evidence of being self-centered, and my oral delights will not be received with the utmost gratitude. Gratitude is key if it's to be a regular thing. (Not because I'm bent on being worshiped, but because it's such an intimate, intense exchange! I'm practically weepy with gratitude after I come from pussy-licking!)

I never had an orgasm from doing it but I've definitely gotten hot and wet.

This is for guys who can't convince their gals to give them blow jobs. If you're making out and in the nude, slowly move your body up so your penis is touching her breasts. Then take your penis in hand and start rubbing the head against her nipples. If you have pre-cum going, so much the better. I've found that BJ-shy women are so turned on by this that it is very difficult for them to resist at least kissing the penis. Once they have done that, then they are apt to continue. I think the main point is that you make it her decision, not yours, to do the blow job. By presenting your penis to her in such an erotic fashion, it helps her to let down her guard, and then make the decision to go ahead if she wants to.

———

No teeth. Don't stop. Keep your hair out of the way. Change things around after a couple minutes. Lick the head like a lollipop. Act like it is your favorite toy in the whole world.

———

Don't neglect his balls, though! I like fingertips and/or nails to lightly stroke my scrotum while my cock is being devoured. Lips and tongue migrating down there every once in a while don't hurt my feelings none, neither. Just remember to keep it light.

———

Maybe we should let them in on the secret that just because they are called "balls" doesn't mean they're really like balls ... more like boiled eggs? Really *sensitive* boiled eggs.

———

If you're into rimming, some back-and-forth action between north and south can be enjoyable.

———

Do it like you mean it and enjoy it. The worst BJ in the world is when the woman acts like she's just doing it because the guy wants it!

———

For me ... it's all about enthusiasm ... that's all it takes.

———

It doesn't have to be perfect for it to be good. You don't have to be a porn-star fellatrix for him to enjoy it. Do what you enjoy, get into it, and he'll love the experience all the more for your enthusiasm.

———

Contrary to popular belief, it's not always great being a man: We die earlier, we don't stand a chance in divorce court, and getting laid is not always as easy as one would like it to be. However, Nature did even the score: Beer, football, women, boxing, fast cars, standing when we pee, and *blow jobs!*

CHAPTER 10

Anal Play

I t is a popular belief that all gay males enjoy anal stimulation and that no one else—straight men or women of any flavor—does. There are also the common assumptions that anal stimulation equals anal intercourse and that anal intercourse hurts. As you can see from the following, none of these beliefs is necessarily true. In some cases, the writer's sex is made apparent by the mention of her clitoris or his prostate. In some cases you can't tell who is doing what to whom beyond the fact that someone's anus is happily involved in the goings on. Good. That only serves to demonstrate the range of anal play enjoyed by men and women of all ages and types.

Begin a process of self-exploration so that you know what goes on down there. By inserting one well-lubed finger you can actually feel your sphincter muscles relax and contract at will. When you are sexually aroused they tend to relax more easily. Work up to two fingers over a period of days or weeks. In general, when he can easily insert two fingers then his erection will likely fit, unless he is thicker than average.

———

Approach anal sex from the point of view that it should be done for your pleasure! If the two of you can find ways to pleasurably stimulate you anally, then anal sex and anal play will become pleasurable and fun.

———

Use a series of progressively larger anal toys. Start off with a small butt plug, one the width of a finger. As much as I enjoy anal sex, having regular intercourse while wearing a butt plug is also extremely pleasurable!

———

Some men don't have a clue as to how to have anal sex. They are too rough, forget they are inside someone else's body. For those who do care about their partners and take their time it can be a wonderful thing, although I have yet to come just from anal penetration.

———

Here's what is for me—those crazy nerves. I don't need a lot of penetration, I don't really need any penetration, although it does feel nice. But I do love the way the head of his cock pushes against my anus and I can feel that taut muscle start to spread itself. It feels tremendous. And then the way those same muscles close tight as soon as his head is in and really grip his cock as he slides further in. I'm much more aware of the grip my anus has on his cock than the grip my vagina has on it. For him, I think it is about the "naughtiness" of the act. I think he *likes* to have a girlfriend whose ass he can fuck. I think he likes having a finger in my puss and a finger in my anus because it's a switch from the norm. I think he could learn to really enjoy it for the tightness and the heat. If you're comfortable with your partner and you're curious, give it a go. If not, don't. It's very nice, but it's not something to try unless the desire is there.

About condom use and anal sex: If you are a monogamous couple, there is a very small risk of a urinary tract infection to the man. If you are not a monogamous couple, there are serious disease risks for both partners. Here's what the Stop AIDS Project says, in part, about the anus: "Your ass is more delicate than most parts of your body. Putting things, whether a finger, cock, dildo, fist, or zucchini, up your ass can tear the lining. Even extremely small tears or scrapes provides a route into your bloodstream. HIV and other STDs can get in or out." In sum, if you're not long-term exclusive, you must wear a condom. If you are, wear a condom if cleanliness is an issue for you. With a female partner, it is imperative that you do not switch between the vagina and anus without using different condoms or completely washing the penis. The vagina is very susceptible to infection.

Some men seem to worry about getting feces on their penises with anal sex. As an ass man, a gay top man who lives by the adage "If it ain't anal it ain't sex," I have topped dozens of men and had regular anal intercourse with my lover. My penis gets feces on it less than 10 percent of the time. None of the men used enemas or lower bowel rinses or waited until after a bowel movement. I think body position-ing might have something to do with it. If the receiver is on his (or her) back, knees to chest and butt pointing to the ceiling—no feces. If the receiver is on all fours—no feces. If the receiver sits on it—some-times feces. It's probably a gravity thing.

Anal beads: It has been my experience that it takes some practice to use them well. The most effective use is to pull them out during orgasm. That's quite a trick to accomplish since the anal muscles usually tighten up at that time. Suggestions—use plenty of lube, make sure they are clean (don't use the same beads on more than one person or go between rectum and vagina), take your time, and experiment. One good method is slowly pulling out the beads from her rectum while you are licking her clitoris.

———

I love everything about the anus. I enjoy anal sex, anilingus, and just plain touching and poking. I also enjoy receiving everything I just mentioned. When I used to masturbate as an adolescent I enjoyed touching that area and inserting things (like the end of a hairbrush). It was never something I had to be taught, and I never viewed it as disgusting. My wife, on the other hand, hangs out in the opposite camp. She permits touching, but has asked—and I've complied—that anal sex for her be a thing of the past. She's willing to do anything to me I ask, and believe me, I do ask! We were having anal sex at least weekly, and she seemed to be more relaxed about it. We started reading *Anal Pleasure & Health* by Jack Morin, and she had several "aha's" and I was excited about future prospects. Then we got to a point in the book where he says that anal sex is also known as *sodomy!* Whoa! That did it! Sodomy is illegal, stirs up memories of the sins of Sodom and Gomorrah, and is profoundly homosexual. The book has been closed ever since. No anal sex.

———

I had a girlfriend who introduced it to me, and it was the first time I experienced a multiple orgasm. We were going 69, and when I was about to come she probed my anus as I was coming.

———

About two months ago I was treated to a very unusual surprise, albeit a pleasant one. One night my wife was feeling particularly amorous and asked me to lie on my back, close my eyes, and just relax. I was very relaxed that night. Anyway the next thing I know she has me spread my legs and cups her fingers in a point just below my ass. Then she pours a very liberal amount of liquid lube (Astroglide) on my balls and lets it run down between my legs and dams it in her hand over my ass. She then inserts her finger into my ass and with it went most of the lube. By this time I was extremely aroused; she cooed to relax and wait so I did, and before I knew it she had four fingers in my ass up to her knuckles. She asked me if I wanted more and she folded over her thumb and put that in too. Boy, what a rush! She began to slowly move her hand in and out up to her knuckles. After a short time she rotated her hand slowly and, to my surprise, popped right inside. Oh! My! I almost came right there. Then she grabbed my cock with her other hand and put it in her mouth. That was it for me. So all you husbands and boyfriends out there, if you can overcome your inhibitions about anal penetration and not see it as unmasculine or something that only gay men do, you are in for a real big treat. That must have been the most intense orgasm of my life, no lie.

You can use a variety of products that contain benzocaine—Anal-eze, Maintain, and so on. They help the sphincter muscles relax. A small vibrator also helps. You might try controlling the action as well. Sit astride him. Or spoon. Start off slow and easy. Go for a few minutes, clean up, and continue with a different activity. Give yourself a chance to become accustomed to it. Save the wild anal escapades for when you are both truly ready!

I enjoy anal sex, and that is largely due to the patience and sensitivity my S.O. has for me. If he is going in and I tighten up, he stops pushing and gives me a moment to relax. He even asks if he's hurting me if I give the slightest signal that it might be. We like anal sex, but we don't indulge in it all of the time, so we still have a bit of a time getting his penis in. But once it's in. . . .

There is this thing he does to make my anus relax. He takes the tip of his dick and rubs my hole with it. That tends to feel like a tongue licking it.

I want to second the motion on Astroglide. For any kind of anal penetration I find it's far, far better than K-Y Jelly. (Indeed, it's better for everything, really—hand jobs and vaginal sex too. I wonder why K-Y is still so popular?) My girlfriend and I had a pretty tough time getting her to relax enough for anal sex, but when we tried using Astroglide instead of K-Y, suddenly everything clicked quite nicely. You do have to use a lot of it, though.

———

When I had my first prostate exam, man, it hurt like hell. Then the doctor told me this little secret and it seems to work. The one trick about relaxing the anal muscle is for the receiver to push "out" as if she were going to the bathroom. Because the anus feels invaded, it tends to contract, and that's when it hurts. Anilingus works wonders, and also when the receiver is very hot it helps to relax. Start with the fingers. Go easy. One finger first, then two, and you'll see the possibilities. But she has to be open-minded to it, don't force her. Once you know how to do it, it doesn't really hurt. Careful, the inner walls of the rectum are very sensitive.

———

I don't know why there are so many hang-ups out there about anal sex. It's not kinky. It's not weird. It doesn't hurt. It's not any more dangerous than vaginal penetration. It's just different. When I first tried it, it was wonderful. I think a lot of men are more open to it because they have that thing-a-ma-gig that is like a divining rod and just wants to fit into anything that it possibly can. Instructions are quite simple really. A woman has to be *very* relaxed. Some women need lots of lubrication. I never did. I usually was wet enough from vaginal stimulation that my lovers could just slip into my anus. A woman does not have to have an enema. Just keep track of your bowel movements. Within twenty-four hours of a bowel movement there's room for him. I really don't like to plan sex *that* much. If you can practice safe vaginal sex without a condom or if you are both monogamous and clean, there's no need to use a condom for anal sex. Just remember that he needs to wash if he's going to penetrate you vaginally again.

———

My husband and I enjoyed anal sex fairly regularly. He was enjoying anal play for a long time before I was ready for it. I stimulated him with my finger and toys. Years into our relationship, we finally had anal sex involving my anus. I really enjoyed the sensation, and since he'd been there before, he knew just how slow to go. When my current sweetie suggested it, I was all for it. His wife had never allowed more than a finger in her anus, and he wanted to know what it was like. Was it tighter? Warmer? This being the one area where I felt more experienced, I was eager to teach him something. He was incredibly turned on to be doing something considered "naughty." We used plenty of lube, I was relaxed and aroused. I thought I was ready, I was guiding his penis in. *It hurt so much I saw stars!* His penis is thicker than anything I'd had in there. For now, we're sticking to toys in the back. Last year's Valentine gift was a graduated butt plug collection (his and hers). Soon, I'll be ready for that anal sex I so desire!

———

Would I do this with my wife if she let me? In a heartbeat! Do *I* think she is missing a great sensation? Absolutely! But she doesn't think so, and the issue is dead. I *never* bring it up anymore. Why should I? Sex is about mutual respect, gratification, and pure trust. For me to keep prodding her (no pun intended) about an act she is fearful of simply destroys the whole idea of mutual bliss. We do everything else, and we do it quite nastily. I am 100 percent fulfilled without anal sex. Oddly, it was an initial request to try it that led to her inserting a finger in my butt. Sent me over the top. That's why I think she is missing something, but that isn't my call. If she wants to try it, she'll have to ask because I won't ask again. I would be devastated if she gave in to me and I caused her great pain. And as for having men try it first. It's a great idea. But I'll tell you this. I like it so much we bought me a vibrator . . . and a good-sized one!

———

I would suggest that you start by letting her just penetrate you with her finger, slowly, taking your time with lots of lube to get you used to the feeling. If you decide you like this and want to buy a strap-on, keep a few pointers in mind: Size is completely your choice but I would start small, giving your anal muscles time to get used to it. Taking it slow is very important, especially in the beginning. If she penetrates you too hard and too deep at once, she has a big chance of hitting your prostate, which can be very painful and not what you're looking for. It also gives you a chance to enjoy the feeling, get used to it, and relax. The more relaxed you are the better it goes. Don't be cheap on the lube, not in quantity or in quality. You don't wanna run dry. So get a lube for anal sex (it's thicker and lasts longer mostly), which might be a bit more pricey but well worth it. Very important! Communicate; tell her what you like, how it feels so she knows she's hitting the right chords. And if it doesn't feel good, just stop and try a bit further the next time.

———

Prostate massage is important to men's health. Bending your boyfriend over is good for him. In fact, he needs it. Just be very slow in your first penetration, use *plenty* of K-Y Jelly, and use a smooth dildo.

———

I am a female, and I totally enjoy it. I have full minute-long orgasms while doing anal sex. It took a lot of time, practice, patience, and trust. You can't just "go at it" the first time and expect everything to be fine. The muscle has to learn to relax—and so does the woman attached to it! Any position where she can be relaxed is cool. You might want to try to work up to it through oral sex. It relaxes everything, and you could move to anilingus. (Have you tried anilingus? Some people don't even realize how sensitive and erotic that area is!)

———

I would suggest that you explore the topic together. Read up on the health issues, find some good quality erotic stories that feature anal sex as a theme, rent or purchase some good quality porn that includes anal sex. It is OK to admit to your lover that this turns you on, but do not make her feel obligated or guilty. If she decides she does want to experiment, do it on her timetable and let her call the shots. Be patient, thoughtful, and loving. This is an act that requires a lot of trust. Use a good lubricant. I prefer the ones specifically formulated for anal sex. Use lots of it, on you and her, inside and out. Prepare her for penetration by inserting a finger, then two, and when penetrating, go very slowly. It is the initial entry that is most difficult and most likely to cause pain. Let her set the pace of your thrusting and depth of penetration once you get in.

———

The first time I tried it was with my ex-husband; it hurt a lot and I finally had to disengage. (He never got past the head.) He was petulant and pouting about my inability to take it all the way, and I *never* allowed him to try again. The way he handled it really repressed me sexually for the remainder of our marriage and made me much less inclined to try new things overall. It took me several years after our divorce and a very caring lover to try it again. It worked out and I became orgasmic during anal sex after a few tries. It became a fairly regular part of our sex life.

———

I have found saliva to be an excellent lubricant. Two of my lovers perform fellatio first and then have me enter their recta. Both say that performing fellatio causes the anal sphincter to relax and respond wonderfully to anal sex.

———

Anal play is not limited only to penetration. If he's down on me, all he has to do is rub the outside of my anus with a fingertip or knuckle and I'm putty. The anus is just too packed with nerves for it not to be enjoyable.

———

My girlfriend made a great discovery for me. Without telling me, during 69 she would caress very gently around the opening of my anus and also the inner part of my cheeks. It felt so good. She did a little fingering and I did not even realize it, I was having such a great time.

She'd also roll up a tissue paper to be pointed, and would very gently caress my anal opening. It feels so good. I guess there's nothing wrong with getting to know all your erotic parts.

My girlfriend is very orgasmic during anal sex. There should be little pain if you know how to penetrate.

I've never heard of anal sex causing constipation. This is one of those areas where once in a while, people may mistakenly assume a cause-and-effect relationship when there is none—a person has anal sex and wakes up in the morning constipated, then assumes the anal sex caused it, when in fact it was brought on by more common causes such as lack of fluids or diet. It's also probably an example of the forbidden fruit theory. Anal sex is thought by many people to taboo, and various "old wives' tales" are built up around the practice—like you will get constipated or you will get hemorrhoids or you will (fill in the blank). Education and enlightenment are the keys to debunking these false myths.

The enema in advance doesn't make a bit of difference other than to get my gut all knotted up, which is a good way to get me out of the mood, so I tend to skip that step and just wash real well instead.

It started as something I wanted to do for my significant other. In fact, each time it usually starts that way, but now I really like it. It's a combination of things, maybe one is significantly more important than the others: it's taboo. That gets me going. As to the pain, that's not a great aspect, but my S.O. is *very* considerate. So when I say slow down, he does. (If I wanted pain, I'd get a spanking.) It serves him well, because if he forced it, he'd be outta there.

I like nothing better than looking through my legs (up on his shoulders) to his face when he's coming up my ass. Delicious! Apply a finger to my clit and I'm right there with him!

Supposedly it's one of the best ways to stimulate the G-spot because of the natural downward pressure of the cock head when you're in there, so that could account for some of a woman's enjoyment.

It's not something I've ever suggested to a partner, but I have been with some who didn't just suggest it, they were passionate about it. They *really* got off on it, and I, for one, love it when my partner has enough self-confidence to suggest something she is passionate about. Surprisingly, there didn't seem to be a pain factor involved, but obviously they had been experienced with it in the past.

In the beginning there is some discomfort, but with a gentle, considerate partner and lots of lube in can be minimal. It also gets better with time! I'm glad I didn't stop having vaginal sex because it hurt the first few times!

The best part about it is if the guy will make love to my ass before, licking, tonguing, rimming with his fingers and mouth. This usually gets me hot enough to where I've got to have something penetrating somewhere, and if he loves my ass, let's do it!

Try having him stimulate your anal region with gentle massage while he sucks and licks your clit. After a long while, when he is fully excited have him insert an anal plug with a built-in vibrator slowly into your anus. Turn the vibration way up. Have him climb aboard and enter your vagina with his rock-hard penis. The anal plug will vibrate the sensitive underside of his penis through the vaginal wall. Guaranteed to give both of you a mind-blowing orgasm.

I have to tell you that enemas cause me to have mind-blowing orgasms. It's not something that I do very often, but I'll explain how it works—and what it does for me. I do this with my wife's assistance, but there's no reason that the same thing wouldn't work as a masturbatory experience. Enemas work by stimulating peristaltic action in the intestines. That's a muscular contraction that runs the length of the intestinal tract, with the effect to push out or void any material in the way. Peristaltic action is like a series of waves, one contraction right after the other. In order to stimulate the peristaltic action, there must be some mild irritant in the enema. I generally use a standard bag with a bit of liquid castile soap. I happen to use Dr. Bronner's. Once the enema is injected, you must hold the solution for a time (five or ten minutes) for the peristaltic action to begin. I prefer to try to hold it as long as possible. In the meantime, you stimulate yourself toward orgasm. For me the payoff comes when I reach climax. I lose control. That is to say that I can no longer hold in the enema. I give in to the peristaltic waves. Everything goes on autopilot. Specifically, I have an orgasmic contraction, followed by an anal contraction expelling part of the enema. The contractions alternate, giving me a tremendously prolonged orgasm. As I love the anal stimulation, I end up in a state that's just hard to explain. If it works, its great; but I can't say that it works for everyone. And be sure you do this someplace appropriate like a bathtub or shower or somewhere else where you're prepared for the clean-up.

———

Learning to relax your sphincter muscles in order to better enjoy anal sex is one way to better bowel health!

CHAPTER 11

Varieties

"One man's meat is another man's poison." There are so many folk expressions that convey the idea that individual preferences differ and that what suits one person will suit another not at all. That's certainly true of most sexual pleasures. What's included in this chapter might be called "creative sex play" by some and by others "kink." Alex Comfort, in his early '70s groundbreaking book *The Joy of Sex,* called such things "pickles and sauces," I believe. Whatever you call it, what's covered here is sex in its more "non-vanilla" aspects, and the comments are purely the opinions of the players.

Two's Company, Three's a Party

Having more than one partner at once, experiencing same-sex contact in a somewhat safe context, and watching one's lover with another person are all common fantasies. A threesome combines them all, so it's not surprising that discussions on this topic are frequent and popular on the Sexuality Forum.

It's impossible to generalize about how easy or difficult it is to arrange a threesome. There was a time when I thought that it was easier to set up a Male/Male/Female threesome rather than an FFM. I thought that many if not most guys would jump at any chance for group sex, even if they had some reservations about the possibility of male homosexual contact. Also, I thought that most threesome-curious straight women would be more comfortable with two guys rather than a gal and a guy. But those were misperceptions on my part. It's really all dependent on the dynamics of the people involved, and I think that just as many women are willing to try threesomes as men.

———

My experience with a threesome was *exciting,* yet underwhelming. It did not involve my S.O., but rather a friend and her sister. While the novelty was noteworthy, something I'll never forget, the actual session was not my cup of tea. I prefer to give and receive intense and focused personal attention during sex, and I found this combination to be very distracting.

———

I can speak from experience that while the fantasy of a threesome might sound exciting, seeing another man intimately involved with your mate and her enjoying it can lead to some tense moments. (For all three of you!) She might have a hard time letting go, for fear of you being jealous, he might have a hard time feeling comfortable, and you might not like it at all, especially after your first orgasm. Once your lust is sated, you might find it upsetting that another man is snuggling your wife and getting ready to have another go at her. On the other hand, you all might just love it! One other caution, my personal experience has been that once you try this, you will eventually try it again, even if the first experience was less than satisfactory. It is a highly charged form of sex that can be pretty alluring for both of you and can lead to other fantasies being acted out. If you don't want to open this door to these possibilities, I'd suggest that you don't start at all.

———

Until you two can sit down and talk frankly and openly and honestly about the concept, then it should remain a fantasy. Talk about how you would feel, the effect it might have on your relationship. Talk about how you would select the third person and the kind of relationship you might have with him or her. Talk about limits and a safe word. Talk about where you'd do it. Talk about STDs and birth control. Generally it's best to know the other person very well. Date him. Socialize with him. Then talk to each other again and again.

———

Condoms are a *must*. Have a basket of them. Change between partners and positions. The only other choice is not to do it. Before you head off to the room, be sure to talk with your partners long enough to get to know who they are.

———

I believe that there are some pretty well-established guidelines for conducting oneself safely in situations when the partner(s) are strangers, someone you met through the Internet or a personal ad. You first meet them in a public place during the day, without any plans for activity; don't give out personal information; if an encounter is arranged, tell a friend where you will be and for how long, and arrange for them to call you at a specific time; and don't include drugs or alcohol in any meeting.

———

As an avowed "multi-tasker," I have had quite a few MMF three-somes, in about half of which the lady had not done it before. The important thing is *your* comfort level going in. You need to know these guys and fully discuss all your concerns well before you jump in the rack together. Take your time setting it up. As a gal looking for one of these things, *you* are in the driver's seat. *You* have the negotiating power. Use it! Insist the guys use condoms. What's OK and what's off limits to you? Are you into oral, anal, would you like to try a double penetration? Tell them about it ahead of time. Again, any hesitation or reluctance expressed on their part and they're out. Don't worry about feeling badly if it turns out these are not the right guys. *You* need to have a comfort level here. And believe me there's no shortage of guys who would *jump* at the opportunity. It's a popular male fantasy, too, although it seems to me that more guys look for the FFM kind of threesome activity. I've had the most fun with people with whom I was acquainted beforehand. Personal ads are a bit risky, I think. It shouldn't be all that difficult to entice some open-minded male acquaintances into this sort of activity. In fact *one* male friend can often scare up another without too much difficulty, and it's a lot better going into one of these things with a friend.

———

There are lots of ways to approach people on the idea of three-somes or other varieties of group sex, and what works best for one person will not necessarily be the best for others. It's a matter of your own personality and preferences. There is, of course, the advertising route, using personal ads in newspapers or on the Internet. Or, if you live in a large urban area like San Francisco or New York, there are sex clubs you can go to where you can seek out people who share your interests. So-called swingers groups exist all over the country, and are another way to link up with people who have poly-sex preferences. These groups are often represented on the Internet, and there are many national and regional swingers' magazines. I favor simply being honest and open with friends and acquaintances, allowing my interests and preference for group sex to be made known during conversation and then gauging their reactions to determine the level of interest or curiosity.

———

One thing for sure is that you don't want to pressure or force anyone into group sex. Some fantasies should remain fantasies. In my personal experience, if you *do* get people to talk about group sex, more people of both sexes are willing to try it than you might imagine. (Maybe it's just the kind of weird people I hang out with.) Certainly, if you are in or getting into a new relationship, your preference or desire to try group sex can have an effect on that relationship. My advice would be to bring up the subject cautiously but persistently. You'll be able to get a reading pretty quickly as to how your partner feels.

———

I have had a number of threesome experiences—some disastrous, some the most divine sex of my life, all with me as the third. In the interest of moving toward this I have found two things quite useful. (1) Talk first and be honest. What does each person want (sexually, emotionally, for the short term and the long term)? What does each person need to feel safe? Are there any limits on who may do what to whom? Are there any specific acts or combinations that would or would not feel good? Starting by building trust and rapport helps to create the space where any one of the three may stop the action if it goes in a direction that doesn't feel good. (2) Commit to being a threesome for your play date, rather than two plus one. Make sure that each person gets some of what she or he wants. This might include some version of pairing off, focusing on one person at a time, or maintaining a balance of attention to all three individuals throughout the session.

Cross-Dressing

A man who wears a skirt could be a Scotsman or a transvestite. Some men dress as women as part of their journey toward becoming women; these are transsexuals. Some men get a great charge out of particular items of women's wear, such as silk panties under their business suits; they are called fetish dressers. For others, dressing in women's clothing is a Halloween event or a one-time playing dress-up experiment. Since there are so many possibilities, a man wearing garments that in his society are understood to belong only to women can have a number of meanings—sexual or non.

I think cross-dressing is just a form of liberation. Why shouldn't a man be able to wear a skirt and not be looked at as a freak? Do you look at a woman in pants as a freak? I have worn skirts and make-up on a couple occasions. Hey, I want to feel pretty too! It lets me feel like I'm breaking out of social conventions and it lets me get closer to my feminine side. And it's just plain fun. Have you ever worn a skirt? It's so light and breezy and loose and free. It feels nice sometimes not to have the little privates all bunched up in on themselves. And besides, a skirt is easy access.

———

I had a relationship for a time several years ago with a man who loved cross-dressing. It was really was a big turn-on for me. He actually not only liked cross-dressing, but he wanted to be my "sex slave." The downside of this relationship, for me anyway, was that he wanted to do the fantasy thing all the time. I wanted a somewhat more conventional relationship with the man, although, once again, this was wild and fun; I just couldn't remain into it all the time.

———

I find gender very sexy. I feel that I'm neither one nor the other, but like a hyena or something, changing all the time. I love men and love men's things; I also love women and women's things. Neither feel like they are exactly *me,* but I don't feel uncomfortable in them either. I like dressing up and looking in the mirror and thinking, "Damn, I'm a hot butch," and I love it when people call me "Sir," but I also like dressing femme and feeling girly and how people react to me in both. Both are exciting.

———

Re: The divorced woman who came out of the bathroom and was upset to find her new boyfriend wearing her underwear: I say give him another chance. I have done this twice as a joke with two different women. Both times we had a good laugh because I looked silly. I am not a cross-dresser, just have a weird sense of humor. I wound up living with the first woman for seven years and have been married for fourteen years to the second one. I sure am glad that my lovers were not as upset as your reader. I hope she has not missed an opportunity for a wonderful relationship.

Anal and Vaginal Fisting

Men can be fisted anally; women can be fisted anally or vaginally. The practice has also been called "hand balling," and it is one that calls for plenty of communication, plenty of lubrication.

Fisting continues to be the biggest turn-on for me. I have found that lying on my back works very well, however, doggie-style certainly does appeal.

———

It's important that she is 100 percent into it. In fisting, the fistee does 95 percent of the work. She must relax, really relax, and be able to trust you. You must go slowly and really pay attention to her. Use your other hand to feel her body, and make certain that she isn't tense. Watch her expressions, listen to her, talk to her. Take lots of time and progress very slowly. Use a rotating motion, with light, but constant, pressure. Water-based lube, thick, like Foreplay. Make sure that you apply lube not only to her, but to your hand and wrist, as well. Once in, just leave it there and let her get used to the feeling. It's very overwhelming!

———

My husband's hand is too large, though he can insert all four fingers to the knuckles. I can insert my own hand, however. We both find that to be very erotic. Use a water-based lubricant. They are easier to clean up. Use a rubber surgical glove. This will make your hand slipperier than your skin. Work at it slowly and gradually over a period of weeks or months, even. Every woman is different. Every hand is different.

———

We've tried fisting a few times, still unsuccessful. All about relaxation. Make sure not to use any medication when doing this, nothing to make you numb. We feel really in touch with each other for several days, even without success. Pretty intimate, isn't it?

———

If you want to try it, don't be scared that it will ruin you for regular genital-to-genital sex. It won't. Kegel exercises will keep you working just fine. I always do them right after a fisting session, and it can make great-feeling aftershocks. As to the actual fisting itself, it was stressed to me that a very very very slow approach was the key to doing it without harm, along with a good lubricant. I like Eros massage oil. We use lots of foreplay to get me excited—including masturbation—and proceed very slowly, over a span of probably ten-plus minutes, going in bit by bit and then retreating, teasingly. The most difficult part, and the part that feels the best too, oddly enough, is the portion of his hand through the base of his thumb. He whispers really hot suggestions, moving in S-L-O-W-L-Y as I zero right in on my clit. He has even sucked my clit while diving in. The split-second sensation of his hand making the full entry into my most intimate area is so electric. I can't even make a word just then, only the most guttural moans of ecstasy. The only part of the whole experience that can be rather touchy is having my cervix touched. It feels great being so filled up, but careless thrusting against the cervix just plain hurts, so go carefully until you know how much depth feels good. My whole vagina throbs with the gentle thrusts of my lover's hand. He loves feeling my response in his hand and not his penis; he says it gives him more opportunity to please me without the intense sensations of penile penetration. I have had wave after wave of amazing orgasms this way, as it allows me to focus on working my clit with both hands. The absolutely best orgasms I ever had were from being dived into this way while bending over. Have fun; go slow. It's worth it.

Take your time. It took my wife and me almost two years before we were successful. Also, try a water-based lubricant. We use Astroglide, which is available at our local pharmacy.

It is exciting to do something new, to push the limits a little. And the feeling I get when he actually penetrates and slides deep inside is *very* nice! To be stretched and filled is quite pleasurable . . . and also visually exciting to look in a mirror and see a huge object filling my rear.

My wife loves it. What I usually do is start with three, then four fingers, then move my hand in and curl the fingers once I'm inside. (This, all by itself, has its own set of effects.) There isn't, for me anyway, an awful lot of in-and-out motion. Not distance-wise, anyway, although there is indeed a whole bunch of moving about on my part. Some of it is just moving my fingers about, some of it is a twisting-type action. Frankly, it's a peculiar feeling, having my fingertips up against her cervix. Maybe sometime I should join her on a trip to the OB/GYN and take a look at what I'm pressing up against.

My gynecologist friend tells me she always tells her interested patients the mnemonic OVA—oral-vaginal-anal—to remember the proper sequence and avoid infection.

Voyeurism and Exhibitionism

Watching and being watched are common fantasies. The pleasure that some people take in seeing the sexual activity of others accounts for the high numbers of pornographic video customers.

My wife and I had a friend photograph us twice. It was really hot and erotic. The second time he even got naked. Although it never went as far as a threesome, it was nice watching his hard-on as I was in her. She was *really* turned on by the exhibitionism of the moment. More so than I ever imagined. In fact, had I known exhibitionist behavior was such a turn-on for her, I would have suggested a photo session for our second or third date!

———

I had a canceled appointment, so I went to the porno movies for kicks. In the audience were a man and woman. They got amorous and I figured they wanted to be watched (not that uncommon). She is working on her man when a number of other men come around and begin touching her. Then he gets up and leaves after she assures him she is OK, and she begins having all kinds of sex with everyone who will join. She said it was a fantasy she wanted to live out. This lady spoke articulately to the men around her (as I said, I was right there watching), and it was obvious she was intelligent. It was incredibly hot to see, and I saw everything imaginable.

———

For guys at Mardi Gras there's only one area in which to flash. It's the gay end of Bourbon Street. I will note that most men who flash, gay or straight, pull out a limp penis in exchange for some innocuous plastic beads. For me, the exhibitionism is the thrill, and I'm not limp when I "show."

———

I think it is highly pleasurable and erotic to watch a lady urinate! Why? Because of the sense of intimacy involved, the combined look of embarrassment and sexiness on her face as she is emptying her bladder! I just find it so sexually stimulating to watch that combined look of embarrassment and coyness.

Watching a female pee is a tremendous sensual experience. The sight, sound, smell, and feel are all-powerful reminders of our wonderful animal nature; there is a very human essence in pee. Don't forget that animals mark their territory (or their mate) by peeing.

A very recent fantasy involved a meeting of the board of a community service organization. Budget issues were being discussed, and the meeting tone was almost somber. In my fantasy, I place myself in the open area surrounded by eight men and three women seated at tables. Music begins playing, and I do a slow striptease. The other women join me, and we move around to each of the men, helping them to "loosen up."

Power Play

There is an alphabet soup of terms covered here: S & M (Sadism and Masochism), B & D (Bondage and Discipline), D & S (Dominance and Submission), as well as activities ranging from piercing to "Lie back and enjoy because I'm taking over for a while." What differentiates some of these doings from those in awful newspaper headlines is that sexual power play is between *consenting* adults and, whatever it may look like, the purpose is the exchange of pleasure.

I go to a "play party" (that's where us kinky folk get together and do things to each other) and accept the invitation of a friend to play.

He cuffs me, attaches my arms to some suspended chains, and flogs me. I get an endorphin rush from this and have a wonderful time. In this situation we are "play partners." He is "topping" me. I am "bottoming" to him. If after some time we date and come to an agreement, he is "the boss," my "dom," and I am now his "sub" (as in dominant and submissive). At this point our relationship is exclusive. I cannot bottom to anyone else without his permission. If we decide on further commitment to each other, we may actually marry or have a ceremony in which he "collars" me. Now he is my Master; I am his Slave. It is important to note here that the word *slave* has a wide variety of meanings, and the power exchange can be confined to the couple's sexual relationship or can extend to all aspects of their lives. It's not quite as demeaning as it may sound. Many masters or mistresses commonly refer to their slaves as their treasure and the most important person in their lives, whom they care for, protect, and love.

The sub needs to establish exactly what his or her limits are. State specifically what you will and won't do, the kinds of fantasies that you want to be forced into. A good dom will run with the suggestions and try to take the sub to the edge of the stated limits (constantly checking in with the sub to see that he or she is OK), and possibly ask for permission to go further. There are several books out about learning to be dominant. Also some books about topping from the bottom. You might check with QSM, a catalog and online bookseller.

I gave my girlfriend of six months frequent orgasms by hand or tongue, but she would not bring me off "just yet." Instead she enjoyed massaging my genitals with baby oil, keeping me turned on and fully erect all weekend, every weekend. She finally let me come, taking me by surprise. I was on my back, on the floor, while she sat with her legs folded, facing me, watching TV, while she very slowly stroked me up and down with baby oil. After a while I got close to the edge so, as usual, I warned her. Normally, she would have eased off at this point until I could gain control, but she ignored me and kept going. I got scared thinking she hadn't heard me, so I yelled at her to stop because I couldn't hold back. Instead, she continued her excruciatingly slow stroking as she smiled and said she wanted to see me come right now. Seconds later I had the most powerful and pleasurable orgasm of my life. After eight months of waiting it blew my mind. Since that day I have come three more times, but I never know when she'll let me. Psychologists say that irregular gratification is an effective training technique, so I guess I've been trained by an expert. I still give her all the orgasms she wants, hoping for my reward. The teasing, torture, and anticipation are more fun for me now, because I know what's in store, though I have no idea when.

I love to watch how much she gets off on doing something I am telling her to do, and I think that's a big part of what makes it good. I'm watching to see what really rocks her, what she likes, and am getting better at telling her what she has to do. I keep adding things to the repertoire, and making her do the things that make her the craziest.

I just finished a book, *Some Women*, edited by Laura Antoniou, which contains forty essays written by women involved in D/S. It was an eye opener, to say the least. Try to find yourself a group; they are everywhere. In Philadelphia I have found a monthly get-together to watch and learn, and its a great place to meet like-minded people.

To the woman who has bondage and discipline fantasies and is willing to forgo these fantasies to have a "normal" relationship: I think she is making a huge mistake. I am a man in my fifties who has had bondage and discipline fantasies since puberty. I've been married for more than twenty-five years, and my wife wouldn't consider exploring B & D. Outside of my sexual frustration, our marriage has been good. I have secretly been to professional dominatrices. The sessions have been sometimes good, sometimes bad. When I have a good session, the feelings of satisfaction, contentment, and fulfillment are far superior to any other feelings. I can't imagine how wonderful it would be to play fantasy games with a regular partner. Even though I have enjoyed a good life, if I had the chance to do it all over again I would trade it all for the possibility of a relationship with a woman who shared my fantasies. Young lady, think twice. Sexual urges can be quite powerful, especially over the course of time. You are what you are sexually. Don't try to suppress it.

———

A second opinion for the woman alarmed by her S/M fantasies: There no is no need to act out. You could enjoy S/M vicariously as a voyeur. First read *The Bottoming Book* by Easton and Liszt to understand the psychology of power. Then maybe you can watch live players having fun at a safe sex club. San Francisco, Washington, D.C., and New York have them. Real power-exchange play, unlike what goes on in porn, is safe, sane, and consensual. If you're in a really large metropolitan area, like S.F., L.A., or N.Y., there are educational organizations that teach classes where you can learn these things firsthand. If you are somewhere else, such as a smaller city, there are organizations that have get-togethers, often called "munches," where you can get help learning the ropes, so to speak. In addition, there are lots of books out there. Basic introductory BDSM books include *SM 101* and *Screw the Roses, Send Me the Thorns.* I'm reasonably certain there are books about specific topics like Japanese Rope Bondage, which is a favorite of many.

———

A good source is QSM, an online and catalog bookseller (*www. qualitysm.com*). They carry pretty much every BDSM book in print. You can call QSM—there is a group of very helpful women who run it—and they will be happy to help you find books tailored to your specific interests. However, even the major chain stores and many small independents stock the generic books like *SM 101.*

———

We tried something new the other night. A few weeks ago we visited a Web site that featured pictures of penis bondage. It was ... intriguing. Some days later I purchased a hank of small nylon rope. I used about three feet to wrap around my husband's erection, leaving the head of his penis free. After teasing him with my tongue and lubed fingertips, I covered his bound cock with a condom and straddled him! *Wow!* Very unique and extremely pleasurable sensations. I've used dildos and vibes with knobby protrusions and nubbly rings, but this was very very different. I had a quick crashing orgasm to start, then started experimenting with all the different ways to slide his bound cock in and out of my pussy. I'm sure the novelty of the situation had a great deal to do with my level of arousal, but I'm looking forward to doing it again!

———

We use nylon straps that Velcro and clip lock. You can find them in most toy shops! They have many attachments that go with them, not just for wrists and ankles. They are strong and comfortable.

———

If you're not hooked on using rope, may I suggest Jane's Bonds from Good Vibrations *(www.goodvibes.com)*. They're wrist and ankle cuffs lined with fake fur that have four to five feet of webbing attached to them to tie to whatever you can. I've used them with several lovers who enjoyed them, and I've enjoyed them when I've been in them too. They're comfortable and easy to use. They cost $28.

———

One safety feature is to keep something to cut the rope with. We keep a pair of rose pruners handy.

———

Here is a wonderful site dedicated to the art of tying knots: *www.geocities.com/Yosemite/2158/index.html*. And this one is animated to demonstrate the most popular knots: *www.mistral.co.uk/ 42brghtn/ knots/42ktmenu.html*. What I like most about using nautical knots is that they are secure, they have a quick release, and they're pretty.

———

Some people love rope bondage, and for them half the fun is creating beautiful knots. For me, I like security and safety. So we use metal chain and spring clips. Chain doesn't stretch. I use four lengths of chain, about four to six feet each. One end encircles a bed leg and is clipped to itself with a spring clip. At the other end, I use a spring clip attached to a ring on a leather (hand or ankle) cuff (restraint). The advantage of spring clips is that they are removable quickly. In a pinch, a sub can maneuver his or her hand to reach the clip and release the bonds. After securing the sub, if something is a little too loose, it's easily adjusted by moving the spring clip up a few links on the chain.

Outside the Box

Some people, events, and activities just defy description. I am delighted that we all don't fit into neat little boxes, aren't you?

Guys, this isn't easy and it requires a good amount of lung power. I thought of how the vagina reacts when a woman is excited, and, apart from the engorging, it actually expands, drawing in air if there's nothing plugging it up. Since it expands when excited, it also gets excited when it expands. One evening during lovemaking, I took an unrolled condom, inserted it into her and blew it up. The pressure alone was enough to send her through the roof. (If you can't find the G-spot, this is guaranteed to hit it.) I blew as hard as I could and held it for as long as I could. To take a breath, I twisted it closed, came up for air, and went back down. I started to blow in and out also (careful not to pass out); this worked great too. Her orgasms came like a machine gun, one after the other, until she couldn't take any more and actually made me stop. If anyone tries this, though, make sure you use a condom and don't blow directly into her. I understand this could cause problems.

CHAPTER 12

Men

I n certain areas of America it is customary for a man to refer to his genitals as his "nature," as in his very essence as a human being, or as his "manhood." What makes a man a man, a human male, is certainly far more than his external sex organs, but it is the most physically distinguishing characteristic.

The Penis

Somehow, I feel there ought to be a fanfare here. *Ta da!* And now, introducing your friend and mine....

There is no portion of my penis that is more sensitive than that little area just behind the head on the bottom side.

———

I personally find flaccid penises kind of silly looking, sort of like a wattle on a turkey!

———

A hard cock is something completely and wonderfully different. "Is that for me?" So much variation too!

———

I'd like to share some of the benefits of a curved or kinked penis (this is assuming it causes neither party any pain or makes intercourse impossible). Oral sex is great, because if I approach from the downward position the curve of my lover's penis meets the roof of my mouth, very pleasurable for him and me. Intercourse is fine. The only problem is entering, with which we need some manual guidance, but once we're joined it is a lovely meeting. I believe lots of loving stroking and acceptance of all parts of our body, whether considered perfect or not, are absolutely the best therapy for any affliction. A lot of "physical" stuff is all in the head, and we can help each other love and accept and enjoy ourselves fully.

Size and Shape

In the all-time Hit Parade of mail and posting subjects, penis size is going to rank very near the top. Our society is particularly crazy-making about the size issue, as it is on sex in general. Men are told that bigger is always better *and* that size doesn't matter. So what's true? Who can you believe? The truth is size does matter ... to some people. To most, it is inconsequential. In any case, since most men are not willing to take the risk of current size enhancing procedures (and rightfully so), a man is better off coming to terms with—and learning how to use well—what he has.

The perfect penis for men and women is nine inches soft, six inches hard. He gets a big one to show off, and she gets a good fit that doesn't hurt.

Small is best! If there are males who feel they need to enlarge their endowment, just read this over and over. Some of us go gaga over a small penis because it's easy to fit the entire organ into one's mouth, give it a massage with the tongue, and possibly fit the testicles in there too. Also, some of us are not equipped to accommodate a large or wide penis anally. I have tried with small-to-large dildos to stretch my anal opening for a year without success. A small penis would be perfect.

No matter what size a guy is, it's a definite turn-off if he's insecure about his dick. I'd rather someone be small and happy with it than any size and obsessing on the subject. Perhaps this is analogous to women who are always asking, "Do I look fat in this dress?"

It's a funny thing, the politically correct answer is, "Size doesn't matter," however (let's face it, girls!), there is a fine-print clause in there. It's like this: As long as it's not too small or too huge.

The wider the dick, the more the muscles are stretched, the more sensation there is. My lover had a very short, *very* wide penis. I had to stretch out all over again until I could take him comfortably. However, once I was stretched out, it felt awesome! I think I stayed with him longer than I should have because I liked his dick.

———

I have had women who were scared away when they found out my size, and I have had women who wanted me for my size. My reaction? I am not a freak show. You want sex you have it with me, not my penis, and if I don't go he don't go either!

———

I have been with one very large man, mostly with average men. Ultimately it's more about his eyes than his size.

———

One thing that strikes me is guys who claim, "I have such-and-such-inch penis and I have not had any complaints." Really, how many women out there actually tell their partner after sex, "That was good, but it would have been better if your penis had another inch or two"?

———

I began using vacuum pumps in my early twenties (I'm now thirty) while dating a woman with a definite preference for the more generously endowed man. At that time I was not lacking, but like many other men, I thought that a few extra inches might be nice. She brought the manual pump home one weekend, and we began to experiment. While in the tube, my penis increased from eight inches to eleven inches according to the markings on the tube. This increase in length lasted for about an hour or so. While the increase in length was nice, the increase in width was astonishing—it appeared to have doubled, and lasted an hour and a half. We used the pump consistently, a couple of times a week, the result being that the increase in both length and width lasted slightly longer each time. Each week my size while erect seemed to be larger without using the pump than it was before the program. It took about four years, but I now have the ten-inch penis I always wanted. The key is to go easy. Only use an electric or manual pump for a few minutes at a time until you have a sense of what you're doing. Pay attention to any hint of discomfort. Bursting a blood vessel as a result of using a vacuum pump is most unpleasant. A final thought: While many men have it in their minds that a big cock is the be-all and end-all of male sexuality, be advised that once you have the dick of your dreams, you may come across Ms. or Mr. Right for whom your pride and joy is just too big. Size queens are not as easy to find as porn videos would have us believe.

Using a vacuum pump, I went from six to eleven inches in the first try, then reduced to about eight inches. I stayed with the program, and in about two months I attained a permanent size of about nine inches long and two and a half inches in diameter. One of my boyfriends went to ten inches and stayed there. There seems to be a limit for each individual. The electric pump is by far the best; suction increase can be obtained by a simple twist of the valves. Of course, the directions must be followed. For the small investment required, I found this penis enlargement method to be well worth it.

It's the whole macho mentality—how much weight they can lift, how much money they make, how expensive a car they drive, how hot a woman they have on their arm, how big a house they live in . . . it goes on and on. And while probably most women don't really care, enough do and make noise about it to send out a mixed message that insecure men pick up on. The only erections other than their own that most straight guys see are in porn films, which doesn't help things either. Guys worried about this are using it as a mask for something else that is really bothering them . . . usually not having a woman, or being in a bad relationship, or worried about not satisfying her sexually. It is easier to blame the penis than to face up to reality about other, real shortcomings in one's life.

I don't think I would receive much argument when I state that the physical aspects of dicks loom large in gay male subculture, of which I am a member. Big hard dicks are grand, both in fantasy and in their absolute here-and-now manifestation. I, on the other hand, am currently having sexual relationships with one man who has a small dick and another man who rarely gets hard. The sex in both relationships is wonderful because (1) we like each other, and (2) both partners and me have sex with our whole bodies. Our dicks are just one area of stimulation. Some other areas are the butt, back, chest, scalp, ears, feet, back of the knees, armpits ... you get the idea. Some body parts that can be used to stimulate those areas, in addition to hands and lips, are tongue, teeth, top of the head. I'm not saying that the sex is great despite a small or flaccid dick. I enjoy their dicks because I can do things with a small hard one or a normal-sized soft one that I cannot do with a big hard one. Unfortunately, I think that most men—gay, straight, and bi—are into their late thirties or beyond before the are able to get off their preoccupation with the physiognomy of their own dicks. I agree with Isadora: Enjoy the dick you've got, as well as the body and person to which it is attached. And if you do, other people will too.

———

My hubby has tried "jelking," also spelled "jelquing." You can look it up using any search engine for specifics. We found it on Yahoo. Seems to be working for him—increased girth as well as length. But then I didn't have any complaints before! Here's a link: *www.ubgonline.com/real_pe101.html.*

———

A guy worries about the size of his penis because he thinks it's of the utmost importance in pleasing a woman (as well as in his inherent right to strut around naked in the locker room). And all the little cues given him by society do nothing but reinforce that belief.

———

Part of the problem is that it just seems (to us guys) that size *should* matter. Guys are a very quantitative species (baseball stats, engine block size), and it stands to reason that a bigger penis will provide more stimulation than a smaller one. Clearly, we're not totally in tune with how females view and experience penetration. Physiologically, sex experts claim again and again that only the first few inches of the vagina are sensitive, and the rest only detects pressure. And many women, probably a substantial majority of experienced ones, will tell us (if we'd stand still and *listen* long enough) that size really doesn't matter much. Emotional commitment, tender intimacy, attending to needs, and technique all outweigh general physical characteristics of the male appendage. But another part of the problem is that there are size queens out there, and they can be quite vocal. The important thing, for us guys, is to realize that size is not an issue or concern for most women. And for the women who *do* like size, most seem to treat it as a "nice-to-have," not a requirement, and would much rather have an average-endowed guy who loves them than a well-endowed guy who's a jerk. Though, to be fair, they probably prefer a well-endowed guy who loves them!

———

I've never cared about how big my dick is, but a lot of women I've met have remarked on it. It's been more of an issue for them than for me, at least to the extent that they talk about it. As long as the woman comes and screams real loud, I don't care what size it is. My tongue does most of the work, anyway.

———

I discovered jelquing and a few other techniques through the Internet a few months back. I have already increased in thickness and in length, and I was already a little above average. Strange connection we men have to our dicks.

———

Until I met my wife and heard her comments, I had no idea how large I was. Never did measure and had no real need to. If size means that much to you, by all means do what you need to do to make it acceptable. I just see no reason to hang a barbell from my Johnson for an extended period of time to accept what I was given. It does what it is designed for, and, apparently, is adequate for the task.

———

I have broken up with women who just couldn't handle my size for any length of time. You can call me a bore, but I usually find a way to let the woman know I'm a super size before things get too far. One way is to invite them to see some photos of me taken at a Halloween party with the warning that the photos have a lot of nudity in them. A nice side benefit of this tactic is that many times I've found myself in bed with the woman the same day she saw the photos. And women claim they're not affected by visual stimulants!

———

Best thing is to run an ad describing yourself as very well hung and find a woman who loves a big one.

———

I have a slender build and my dick is small. I always had some sort of inferiority complex about the size of my dick until I realized that it hardly makes any difference in lovemaking. I am one of the best love-makers (in the word of my ex), and she felt that sex with me was better then anyone else she had earlier. She used to get multi-orgasms from me, which she never did earlier. Be a better learner in the art of pleasing others, and your fingers can do what a twelve-inch dick can't.

———

If a guy's got a big one, he better learn how to use it. It's a sex organ, not a weapon; it's meant to induce pleasure, not harm!

———

If one knows how to use a pea shooter, it can be just as deadly as a cannon!

———

I have some advice for the man who wants to enlarge his scrotum: buy a motorcycle, preferably a rattling, vibrating kind of motorcycle like a scooter or a dirt bike. Unfortunately, I have the problem he wants—a hydrocele, a hard sac of fluid that surrounds a testicle. It's painless, but it's not anything I would wish on anyone. I only have a hydrocele on one side, but perhaps with extensive motorcycle riding or sheer good luck he could have two of them.

Cut or Uncut

This is one sexual issue with wide political implications and medical consequences that are still being debated. Setting those issues aside, if that's possible, what we are discussing here is no more nor no less than personal preference.

I know a man who was circumcised as an adult—a surgeon, single, who has never lacked for impressive female companionship. He assured me that sexual pleasure since the procedure is no different than it had been before. He does not regret that he did it and talks openly about it. I contend that the hands and mouth of a lover encourage me to wallow in the pleasure of his penis skills, regardless of the lack or presence of a foreskin.

My uncircumcised husband is far more sensitive, and oral sex is incredible. Very sexual to see his penis emerge from its shell when he is excited.

The main difference I've noticed between circumcised and uncircumcised men is that circumcised men enjoy stimulation of the glans without discomfort.

I keep seeing this claim that circumcised men are less sensitive than non-circumcised. I don't know where this comes from. I am circumcised, and if I were any more sensitive I couldn't stand it.

The pro-circumcision argument that a boy's penis should look the same as his father's is a hard one to argue with, because it's such a strongly held belief. Yet I think the reality is that *no* little boy's penis looks very similar to his father's. I have this memory as a little boy of urinating with my father. His penis was very different from mine in a variety of ways. It was much bigger, it was a different color (dark brown versus my little pink one), there was a lot of dense black hair all around it, and it was uncircumcised. All in all it looked like a monster. And since I was just a wee tyke at the time, it was right there in front of my face. Had our circumcision status been the same, however, I don't think his penis would have looked any less monstrous to my little boy's eyes.

My new boyfriend is uncircumcised. This is the first time I've ever seen an uncut penis and it is so cute! It looks like a snake in a turtleneck. But when it gets hard, well ... then the head is this massive purple mushroom. Yum!

After carefully exploring all my options, I underwent circumcision at age twenty-two and have been very happy since. If your reader explores this option, he is best off selecting a physician who is both sensitive and artistic to ensure an excellent cosmetic result. I hope he also knows that others will love him for who he is, regardless of circumcision status, and that he need not endure further anguish over an issue for which a meaningful solution exists.

I have had sex with about a hundred men. Two of these were uncircumcised. Of these hundred-plus men, these two stand out in my memory. Why? The sex was better from a woman's point of view—at least this one's. Please urge this young man to reconsider keeping his foreskin. Maybe hearing that some of us women who know what a great thing an uncircumcised penis is and want a man who is uncut will give him more of a sense of appreciation and acceptance for what he's got and who he is.

Me and my roommate are students from France, and we both think it's wonderful that most American and Canadian men are circumcised. Their glans are silky-smooth clean, not sticky and smelly, and the skin along the shaft is tight, not loose, which means they provide much better stimulation for women during lovemaking. It feels exquisite! We wish European societies were similarly disposed toward circumcising their males, and we think someday they will be. Until then, the man who wrote you doesn't need a foreskin; he needs a woman who appreciates his body for the pleasures he offers her.

Erections

Having them when they are wanted and not having them when they are not troubles every man at some point in his life. As for staying power, there are natural-born marathon runners and there are natural-born sprinters (delayed or retarded ejaculators and eager or early ejaculators). Both can learn to modify their styles to suit the game at hand, but as in any behavior modification, it usually takes some not inconsiderable effort. Science (and sexology) are constantly increasing the array of tools to support such efforts.

I have been diabetic for more than thirty years, and one of the challenges is that the vast majority of diabetic men eventually have trouble maintaining an erection. My partner and I have discovered the best solution for us is a rubber ring placed at the base of the penis. Blood goes in, but the ring maintains an erection without any problem. You can buy these by mail order from Encore, Inc. (1-800-221-6603) for about $20 each. Be sure you get a snug fit. Some men need an external vacuum hand pump, which creates an erection by pulling blood into the penis before putting on the ring. One is available by mail order with prescription by Osbon Medical Systems (1-800-438-8592) for about $400. You might also mention the nonprofit Impotence Institute of America (what a name!), which has much information about this challenge (1-800-669-1603).

To last longer, try this Web site: *kinkysexacts.com/premature_ ejaculation/main.htm.* (Why the cheesy title for their Web page, I don't know, but it contains good information on the squeeze technique, breathing, and other valuable information.)

———

Recently someone wrote that her man's penis seemed to have grown larger since their relationship began. You theorized that he might have lost weight, with less belly giving the impression of more dick. Perhaps the fellow was never fully erect when they started. I was a bashful youth and a virgin until the age of twenty-two. The first time I had sex I was overcome by embarrassment and lost any semblance of a hard-on. The next few times it was only by keeping my hand nearby for guiding and reinserting that I could continue. After a couple of weeks I gained more confidence. One night I noticed an increase in stiffness. My girlfriend perceived it as a size difference.

———

I had a boyfriend whose erection was on the small side. After two years together, we discovered that what he really enjoys is some cock-and-ball torture-type stuff. When we practiced this, lo! his erection was almost twice the size I had ever seen it before. I think that tapping into his deeper desires caused the manifestation of a larger erection.

———

Any pleasurable pressure on the groin can cause a man to get an erection. I remember sitting at my desk in high school, and that if I crossed my legs—*sproing!* —instant erection just from the pressure. A man can have an erection even when he has no earthly intention of ever having sex with you. So, when you sit on a man's lap and you feel something, take it as a natural reaction to a pressure that this man's brain does not perceive as unpleasant. If he doesn't have one, that doesn't mean that he thinks you're ugly, simply that whatever criterion his nervous system has for releasing the chemicals associated with erectile function have not been met ... or, that he is capable of enough control to decide not to have one (somewhat unlikely).

———

Men have *no* control over their erections, period, end of story. They happen when they shouldn't, don't happen when they should, and are more or less always a surprise and a miracle, kinda like crocuses blooming in the snow. As a matter of fact, the common phenomenon of men giving names to their penises reflects this strange reality, as personally owning a penis is much like having a bizarre and rabid feral animal joined to you at the hip ... one which has its own desires, its own intentions, its own logic. It does its own thing, like it or not, and damned be the cost. So when someone is nice enough to share his erection with you, always remember that he is almost as surprised as you are, and act accordingly.

———

I've found that I last longer when I'm having sex often, like three or four times a week. I avoid highly stimulating positions. I take breaks from intercourse when I start getting highly aroused. These breaks include various foreplay techniques; I don't smoke a cigarette then start back in. The squeeze technique (outlined in most sex books) was what got me started in endurance sex.

———

For some reason most men just quit after they come. Probably because they think they're done and just give up out of a lack of interest. I discovered long ago that after coming, just keep going in a very slow way, pumping in and out but really slowly, and enjoy every sensation. If you give yourself the time to explore, touch, caress, and find all the wonders of your partner's body and erotic responses while keeping a soft gentle stimulation you will stay hard until the fires reignite, and then it's on to the races. The secret for men and women both is to realize that it's the soft, erotic, gentle caressing and teasing that keeps a man hard after coming.

———

While you are humping, think of sports. Seriously. When you feel yourself about to come, slow down, back off, withdraw, work on ways of stimulating your girlfriend other than through penetration. Then when she has been satisfied or has been brought to the brink you can join back in and have a well-timed dual orgasm.

***

With me, I'd say it depends on how long it's been since the last time, how excited both myself and my lover are, how we're doing it, and how many times we're doing it in one lovemaking session. First times tend to be the shortest if we just plunge ahead (which is what my girlfriend wants at times) rather than playing some delightful delaying games. Five to less than ten minutes seems about average time for me. Further rounds tend to last longer, but again that all depends on how we're doing it. Vigorous, energetic intercourse in a highly stimulating position will always have me coming quicker then a slow and easy ride. Anyway, we usually like to build up close to my peak and then pull back, so that things can last longer.

***

If you come multiple times, the second and third times are usually more relaxed, and you may last longer.

***

A simple and effective method of lasting longer is to apply desensitizing cream onto your glans before sex. However, the cream makes your penis lose some sensation, with reduced pleasure to you, but it does increase your lasting power. Apply the cream about half an hour before intercourse, leave the cream on your glans for only two to four minutes, and then wash your penis thoroughly with water. Wait for half an hour to let the cream's numbing effect fade away, and then have sex. This way, you may retain most of your sensation and sexual pleasure.

***

Viagra seems to have a longer lasting effect than we thought, so that the next day he has no problem with erections. We have both wondered if it's just the relief of being able to sustain an erection that has removed the stress and fear of failure, and that is what is at work here. Whatever it is ... we like it! He is able to stay erect longer with Viagra, and he can maintain it somewhat after he has come so that intercourse can proceed if we wish.

———

You can train yourself to delay ejaculation by many different means. Tantric sex manuals are helpful to many, and more Western-style techniques are taught in many other books that are readily available anywhere. Train yourself to "delay gratification" by taking yourself to the brink of orgasm and then stopping, over and over, and you will gradually develop a sense of when you need to slow down or stop until your responses have quieted down a bit. Then you can proceed.

———

If a woman comes rapidly, I will come very fast too. If a woman keeps going and going, I too will keep going and going. At the first sign that a woman is coming, I too will come. If a woman has a hard time getting to climax, I will put off my climax to try and match hers. The problem is if I put off coming too long, I lose the frantic desire to come. It becomes a quest to thrust as long and as hard as I can. The whole thing ends in an anticlimax. In the end I can't come at all. It no longer was a pleasurable experience, but a quest to see if I can get the woman to climax. Usually, both of us fail, and it leaves both of feeling empty and unfulfilled.

———

A lot of time longer intercourse may be achieved by longer fore-play (oral, petting, necking). This has really worked for me and my wife. You are able to build a resistance to being overcome with the urge to orgasm yourself. If you and your mate are into it, I really suggest lots of oral sex to get both of you to a more longer lasting state of mind. Even if she is not into oral sex, you may still be able to promote your ability to last longer just by servicing her orally for extended periods of time.

———

Orgasms and Ejaculating

In some societies the separation of these two events is an achievement to be prized as an aid in conserving precious male energy, as well as for birth control and for pleasure. For most men in Western society, these two events are simultaneous, as you can see by the language often used here. Their separation can be learned ... with effort.

The tricky thing is to learn to separate the sensations of orgasm from the sensations of ejaculation. Not many men have the patience to learn it, but it's definitely possible. One of my former housemates taught himself to do it as a teenager, because he didn't want to make a mess that his mom would find. Later in life it turned out to be a useful talent in other ways.

———

I've had actual multiple orgasms—orgasms with no refractory period between them, something like one every ten to fifteen seconds or so. For the first time last night I had two orgasms in a row, same as above, except I didn't stop stimulating myself. It was probably a special case, though, since the timeline would have looked something like this (time listed in seconds):

$t - 5$—point of no return reached, stopped stimulating member

$t - 4$—stimulated prostate

$t + 0$—ejaculated, tiny orgasm sensations

$t + 3$—began stroking myself, orgasm occurred in full force immediately (had to stop stimulating prostate to do so, was using a little toy for that)

$t + 8$—second orgasm swung up out of nowhere and hit me right as the first was beginning to subside

$t + 15$—stopped

I would say that it was a continuous orgasm, but my impression is that there aren't discrete exclamation points within that orgasm. Then there are the regular orgasms; I'm not sure how many I've had in one day, but it might be upward of six to nine or so.

———

In your answer to the guy who ejaculates too quickly, you might have included methods of having an orgasm without an ejaculation. One benefit is that there is *no* recovery period. Two sources of information on this are (1) the Tantric-based method of Margot Anand's book *The Art of Sexual Ecstasy,* and (2) Taoist-based method of Chia and Arana—*The MultiOrgasmic Man.* Orgasm without ejaculation is accomplished using one's breath, consciousness, and attunement to body energy—no medications.

———

I am a thirty-three-year-old gay man, and I don't always ejaculate for the simple reason that as I've grown older, I realize that I can have a full, complete, and satisfying sexual experience without ejaculation. Like penis size, I think men put too much emphasis on ejaculation. Just lighten up and enjoy the ride.

———

It's possible that on at least some occasions not coming may be a response to allergies. With me, it has become clear over the years that my reaching orgasm is affected by whatever pollens or allergens are in the air. I find, though, that the absence of orgasm can be a fine means of enhancing sexual experience. Duration means better opportunity to move through different positions and is also a good reason for setting aside more time for sex. A couple of my lovers have expressed uneasiness with my not coming, as if that somehow reflected on them, and one was startled when I told her that I didn't need to come to have good sex. For my part, it's simply a source of variety.

———

I've experienced orgasms that seem to last forever. They start building up and building up and, man, it's just like going to heaven and staying there for a while, and it's beyond description. The normal orgasms are great, but when you can prolong them, they are just a blast. I've had a few of them.

―――

The more orgasms you have, the less cum you will have. You can temporarily increase the volume by arousing yourself near to the point of orgasm, then stopping. Do this several times over a period of several hours. Diet can affect volume. Drink lots more water. This seems to slightly increase volume, or at least make it look like more.

―――

The woman making noises and squirming has always brought upon a stronger orgasm, but that doesn't mean I couldn't have a really intense one making love quietly, feeling her breath on my neck, and the electricity of her hands on my chest as we come, staring into each other's eyes.

―――

What happens when you have an orgasm is that fluids from the prostate and fluids from the seminal vesicle mix, and then shoot out, and a chemical reaction has formed. It is white because it is congealed, much the way that blood coagulates.

―――

If I have not come for a few days, my cum is whiter and thicker. I jerked off six times today, and it's very watery and clear.

―――

Just inserting your finger won't make him spurt. You need to apply pressure to the prostate gland. Do this by bending your finger slightly, so that the tip presses toward the front of his body, toward the scrotum and base of the penis. This will put pressure on the prostate. Maintain *gentle* pressure while masturbating him or during intercourse, and he will have not only a mind-blowing orgasm, but also a very copious ejaculation.

―――

Some women do actually enjoy "facials." It's an incredibly intense, erotic, and visual act between lovers. To lie trapped between his thighs as he masturbates mere inches from my face, my hair firmly grasped in one hand, tilting my head back slightly as he spurts hot cum into my waiting mouth and all over my face and breasts . . . ahhhh . . . heaven! I'll never understand where the odd concept of "degradation" comes from with respect to this act. It's no different really than traditional oral sex that ends in the swallowing of the entire amount of ejaculate. It's simply an enjoyable variation, one I even beg for from time to time.

———

I love the way it feels on my face, chin, neck, chest, and in my mouth! What is the difference if he comes in your mouth or around it?

———

My favorite part is when he takes his hands and rubs it into my skin. It feels great! Can't understand what is so degrading about something that both people enjoy!

———

He can come anywhere

In my hair, I don't care . . .

He can come in my throat

Or write cum-notes

On skin

On toes

On my chin and nose . . .

He can come in the air

and watch it land there . . .

On bum

On clit

On breasts and lips . . .

He can come deep inside
While I ride
and slide
Or he can come on my thighs
I don't care . . . *anywhere!*

———

According to my personal experience, the best orgasm happens when you take a long time to get it—get near it, then stop, doing it several times . . . at least ten times, and then ejaculate.

———

To increase ejaculate, drink more water. The second part of the equation is to have a prolonged period of foreplay, culminating in a near-orgasm, as near as you can get. Take your time about it, if possible. Really draw it out.

———

We call it "riding the wave." Let yourself get really close to orgasm and stay there if you can. Back off before you come, and slowly work your way back up, again and again. Fluid intake is important. I doubt that any herbal extracts would help with the volume.

———

I had the most intense orgasm ever the other night. The orgasm was in response to my wife giving me oral sex while in the 69 position. Instead of multiple contractions and squirts, it began with one, and upon the next contraction it was if I was stuck in the "on position." It became one long intense contraction so intense, I literally couldn't breath and nearly passed out. Ain't life grand, just when you think you've done or had it all . . . it just keeps getting better.

CHAPTER 13

Women

I t was not that many years ago that women learned about their sex mostly from husbands and male doctors. The women's liberation movement of the 1970s validated and increased the passing of vital information directly from woman to woman. These days old wives' tales—the kind that transmit women's wisdom and truths rather than rumor and myth—can be young women's, older women's, single women's, the personal reports of all women. Ignorance about our bodies and our sexuality is no longer viewed as a sign of virtue, but simply what it is—ignorance.

Anatomy

Female plumbing has always been mysterious. (Has anyone ever been able to decipher the diagram that comes with a packet of tampons?) Female problems were once attributed to a wandering womb! And today there are ranging controversies about the existence of the G-spot and female ejaculation and even how far the clitoris extends beyond the visible penis-like nubbin. If the experts are not in agreement, the lay opinions (no pun intended) are varied indeed.

The clitoris is on the outside of the body, not in the vagina where the G-spot is.

Your wife has a couple sets of fleshy "lips" (labia) between her legs. The outer ones are often hair-covered (unless she shaves), the inner ones form an upside-down V($\wedge$). That top point, where the legs of the $\wedge$ meet, is where the clitoris is located. It should feel like a little bump buried in the folds of skin that make up the labia. Some women have large, protruding clits, other women have small ones, sort of like penis size—it varies. Usually when a woman is aroused, the clitoris is engorged with blood and becomes more prominent. It also becomes more sensitive during arousal. For some women, touching it is like touching a raw nerve, and they prefer to touch around it. Usually rubbing it in a circular motion (on or around) is very arousing (at least for me). Her response to your touching of it should guide you as to whether you need to go harder and faster or slower and softer.

OK, imagine holding an empty can of Pringles chips in your hand with the opening facing you. Lower it. Got the visual? OK, the very bottom of the can is the cervix and the opening of the can is ... well, the opening. Now, imagine where the clitoris would be placed in relation to the opening. Next, bear in mind that only the very tip of the clitoris extends from the body; the remainder runs like a root a further three to five inches into the body, right along the top of that Pringles can. Kootchie-kootch that root in the right spot and you're going to produce some pleasurable sensations. For some women this might be in the region of the G-spot, for others it might be a bit deeper, say in this cul-de-sac area.

—————

I think we are all just plain different in what excites us. I have a very pleasurable reaction to G-spot stimulation and can orgasm from it. But I can't orgasm from a vibrator against my clit—that hurts. I have to have a soft touch or oral stimulation to come. My G-spot isn't that far inside, maybe two inches or so, on the upper wall of my vagina. If your lover is facing you, imagine his or her fingers hooked in a come hither motion. It usually works best for me if he uses just one finger, his middle finger, and rubs firmly. At first, all I wanted to do was pee and I would make him stop, but now I hang in there and that's when it gets really good, especially if you combine it with oral or manual stimulation of your clit. We're all so different. I have discussed this with many friends, and only one of them has the reaction I do to G-spot stimulation. Others don't like it and the rest haven't ever found it.

—————

I've looked for my G-spot, really I have. We've tried, numerous times, but to no avail. I like to be penetrated, but don't ever orgasm from that alone. There is no spot inside me that feels different from the rest, pleasurable or painful. I don't doubt that other women have them (my partner included), but I don't think it's a universal thing. I've been with other women who don't have them either. I don't think we're malfunctioning. I have great clitoral orgasms and that's enough for me!

—————

In all of my many experiences (two!), one lady received her orgasm from her clit while apparently having no G-spot, while the second lady had little response from her clit but went into ecstasy from her G-spot.

—————

I found the index and middle finger "hook'" on the G-spot accompanied with clitoris kissing makes my baby wild. I also find her gushing cum at this time. I then take my other index finger and flick her clitoris while I move my tongue into her vagina with my fingers. Delicious!

———

I can orgasm from G-spot or clitoral stimulation, but both together is absolutely earth shattering! Ideally his index and middle fingers are hooked inside me, rubbing firmly on my G-spot, and at the same time he is licking my clit, not too hard or fast . . . just building the tension until I am screaming in ecstasy and my hips are bucking. It is incredibly easy to do multiples this way.

———

I found that when I was pregnant my hormones made my clitoris enlarged—not quite the size of my small fingertip, but definitely a good 50 percent larger. After I had the baby all went back to normal. This happened regardless of the baby's sex. It didn't make sex any more fun; it was kind of less sensitive so I was glad when it returned to normal size again.

———

The clit is one of the most highly sensitive, erogenous areas on a woman's body. Now personally, it is not wonderful for me if my partner touches my clitoris before I am "ready" for that. I prefer for him or her to wait until I am tremendously aroused and "aching" for a touch or a lick. In other words, now that you know where it is, it might pleasure your wife more if you didn't just "go straight for it." Tease her with your fingers, your tongue, and so on. After some lovely, extensive foreplay as she is writhing on the bed, it will feel heavenly for her if you lick and lap at it, and then slip that lovely clit of hers into your mouth.

———

The G-spot feels like one of those old-fashioned washing boards. It feels like ridges. If you slid your finger up inside her, turn it to face the front of her body, then hook your finger and wiggle it like you are telling someone to come here, then you will find her G-spot. Her reaction will tell you when you've found it. G-spot stimulation is also very intense, as is clitoral stimulation, so it's also lovely to prolong the ecstasy by not jamming a finger inside her right away and trying to find it. Take your time; allow her to become incredibly aroused and wet first.

The opening to the urethra, whether in women or in men, is a place where many nerve endings collect. Some people just tune into it, and stimulate themselves with small objects, like Q-tips or bobby pins. The thing to be careful of, like in anal sex, is that any objects inserted there can be lost inside unless there is an attached flange or cord to keep them under control. Emergency room technicians are all too familiar with the "I was just cleaning it out, when whoooops" scenario.

Even though the existence of the G-spot is well documented, many of the experts consider referring to it as a "spot" to be a misnomer. It is merely the part of a gland that surrounds the urethra and can be accessed through the vaginal wall. Why not sell magazines by referring to any part of female genitalia that is somewhat sensitive to stimulus in some women (which I would imagine easily covers every inch of the area) as a spot hyphenated by a capital letter, and tout it as a magic button?

Arousal

Arousal is that stage between *ho-hum* and *uh huh!*, from no interest in sex to intense focused interest just before the moment of orgasm. It's a wide continuum.

I am a thirty-three-year-old female who never had an orgasm with my husband. My doctor recommended a sex therapist whom I went to a half a dozen times. I got to read a lot of books and get in touch with myself. I began to tell my husband that I like to masturbate during sex, and now it really turns him on when I play with myself during intercourse. I also took a liking to X-rated films. Just the idea of watching someone else have sex turns me on. Keep an open mind. Whatever it takes to arouse you and reach orgasm, I'm sure your man would be game.

———

We tend to forget we are chemical beings as much as physical and emotional ones.

———

I have been reading a very interesting book entitled *The Alchemy of Love and Lust*. The author, a noted sex researcher, is earnestly hoping that the chemical underpinnings of our sexual lives are better understood and taken into account when sexual difficulties are encountered. PEA, DHEA, estrogen, testosterone, oxytocin, progesterone, prolactin—the hormonal and chemical mix which gives us sexual drive—is complex and amazing. If there is a fluctuation, whether due to stress, illness, injury, choice of birth control method, menopause, then desire will be altered. Many people don't know this, and go through painful self-critical slumps. A lot of people have marital problems and attend counseling when hormones are actually the culprits. It's impossible to will desire if the chemistry is not there, just as much as it would be to walk if nerves are damaged.

———

I heard something on the radio about a new device for increasing the sexual pleasure of women who experience sexual dysfunction. Millions of dollars have been invested into cures for male impotence, such as Viagra. However, this is one of the first for women. It is a small suction device. The suction cup is placed on the clitoris. It then is used to suck blood into the clitoris, making it engorged and stimulated, thereby making the clitoris more sensitive and helping women to feel pleasure and achieve orgasm. Anyway, my fiancée has been through menopause and suffers from decreased sexual desire. So tonight I used the technique on her, but with my mouth instead of the suction cup.

Instead of the standard licking and sucking during cunnilingus, I simply sucked. I took her clitoris between my lips and sucked as hard as I could, pulling it into my mouth. I held it there for a few minutes sucking it as though I were giving fellatio. Her clitoris soon became red and swollen. When we made love she had a wonderful orgasm, the first in a long time.

───

There is a product on the market called Replens, which is designed for women having a dryness problem due to decreased hormone levels. The benefit is that it is used daily, so that the normal moisture level is maintained rather than using a "one shot" lube! I also suggest carrying around a water bottle wherever you go and sip from it constantly. You'll look like a jock!

───

While it may be safe to see your partner's excitement as a compliment, I would not want to jump to the conclusion that a lack of wetness is an insult or disinterest. It could easily be due to work stress, fatigue, or medication. My strongest compliment to my partner is when he can pique my interest when initially I had no interest in sex.

───

I am almost always wet unless I've just finished my period.

───

Too wet? Yeah, that's like having too much money. I love women who get really wet!

Orgasms

One would think that here is a sexual happening with no ambiguity, but not so. There is still much debate about clitoral versus vaginal orgasms, singles versus multiples, and whether one best way to achieve one at all exists. A rose may be a rose may be a rose, but orgasms also come in a variety of colors and styles.

Since I figured out how my body really did work years ago I have noticed that my orgasms are not only stronger but more frequent and easier to achieve. When I compare my sex now to the sex I was having ten years ago the difference is quite remarkable. The reasons I attribute are better familiarity with my body; self-confidence; more ease in asking my partner for what works; and to a large extent, practice. Can't wait for the next decade of sex.

———

There is a foolproof way to find out whether a woman has had an orgasm. A faker can carry on, thrash about, squeeze her pubic muscles, whatever. But what she cannot do is change the consistency of her vaginal mucus. Prior to orgasm it's slippery. During and after orgasm her mucus becomes stickier.

———

I would like to share the secret of an immediate post-orgasmic kiss. It's been my experience that if the woman's tongue is considerably cooler than yours, you can be sure she was not faking it. If, on the other hand, her tongue is the same temperature as yours, she may very well have faked. I have no idea if this is anatomically or medically true, but after fifty years of wonderful sex experiences I've never heard another person note this temperature phenomenon.

———

I am a thirty-eight-year-old woman and can count on one hand how many orgasms I've had. I consider myself to be your average, normal, everyday person. Those women who have orgasms constantly should consider themselves gifted.

———

I have really long-lasting orgasms while having anal sex. Once it begins, as long as he thrusts at about the same pace and in the same manner, I will continue to climax. I haven't ever measured, but it seems like it could just keep going if I'd let him. Eventually we either shift position a little and I start over or I ask him to climax too!

———

I am a fifty-two-year-old bisexual female who has never had trouble getting orgasms—ten to thirty within ten to fifteen minutes by masturbation. Since entering menopause it now takes longer to get orgasms, but they are much more intense and I'm satisfied with fewer (three to ten).

———

I am not sure if my stronger orgasms have to do with age or not. In my case it's because the children are grown and we have more time to spend in private. That leaves more time to explore and find out what feels best, and that leads to better orgasms in general. I am more informed than I was ten to twenty years ago. There is a great Web site that I discovered a while back about orgasms: *www.geocities.com/~debbie_fox/*.

———

According to the *Kama Sutra* and other religious sexual writings, you should roll your eyes back. Doing this opens a chakra that releases sexual energy and creates a more powerful orgasm, and I can definitely vouch for it.

———

I have had G-spot orgasms, which are incredible. It is possible for me to have an orgasm just from stimulation of the G-spot, but it takes longer and is harder to achieve than when both clit and G-spot are being stimulated. A G-spot orgasm is different for me; it seems to come from within. There is a point just before orgasm when I feel an intense need to urinate, and the contractions are stronger than with a clitoral orgasm. It is a harder orgasm to achieve, but well worth it. A clitoral orgasm is more of a sure thing; the intensity grows more quickly. But the best possible combination of events is both at the same time, especially oral and G-spot at the same time. Talk about explosive orgasms . . . ohmigod!

———

It's my impression that what I call a vaginal orgasm involves the tightening and releasing of the PC muscle, the muscle that you tighten to stop urine flow. For me it causes more internal response and deeper orgasmic contractions, whereas a clitoral orgasm comes solely from stimulating the clitoris with no vaginal contact. This type sends sensations more externally. (This is *very* hard to explain.) As far as "training myself," all I know is that I discovered my PC muscle very early on in masturbation play, and it has always been a part of my sexual activity. I would think that any woman could teach herself to do this by learning to use her PC muscle. It does take practice and concentration.

I think that my clitoral orgasms are more intense and long-lasting, especially when they comes from oral stimulation, but I think that my vaginal orgasms are deeper and somehow more satisfying. I think that vaginal orgasms happen more during very intense and long-term arousal, and in my mind are a more emotionally fulfilling experience. Maybe that is connected to the emotional intimacy of intercourse.

For a clitoral orgasm, I need direct clitoral stimulation. A vaginal orgasm I can actually accomplish with *no* manual stimulation at all— simply using internal muscle control—a technique I perfected in college!

I have never experienced orgasm without direct clitoral stimulation. My S.O. and I have found that I have much more intense orgasms through a combination of vaginal and clitoral stimulation in certain positions, but clitoral stimulation is always involved or I don't come.

I *need* more on the clit to have an orgasm. That being said, when he is doing me with his fingers and his tongue and our hips start moving in unison, I'm in heaven. I like both equally, but for me thrusts don't bring about orgasm, sadly.

When I was in my late twenties it felt like I went dead from the waist down, as if overnight. As first it was just that it took longer and longer to orgasm. Later, even if I was aroused out of my mind my vaginal walls were dry, and sex without a lubricant was a thing of the past. I started to use a vaginal moisturizing gel with yam extract, an alternative product supposed to restore a woman's natural lubrication. I don't claim that this is what fixed the problem; it could be just a coincidence that the problems reversed just a few months after I started using it. After three years the seeming clitoral paralysis ended with a bang. My orgasms have become even more intense and easier to come by.

I usually have to be with a man for awhile before I'm able to orgasm. Sometimes it won't happen at all. My BF made me come the first time we were together, and that was an amazing feat. We had a *lot* of chemistry together though, and we had talked a lot beforehand about our preferences.

I have only been able to achieve orgasm by vibrator, water, or as follows: First, I have to consciously relax, exchange kisses and touching. After my partner lightly strokes my clitoris with his tongue I get on top of him in 69 position. I hold onto his bent knees while propping myself up on my elbows. He then continues stimulating my clitoris with his tongue, starting slow so as not to overstimulate. Then he will insert fingers slowly into my vagina and anus (sometimes with the help of K-Y). He continues to use his tongue, and when I am well stimulated he blows on my clitoris like a horn, causing vibration similar to the battery operated vibrator. He interchanges blowing with tongue stroking until I achieve orgasm. As soon as I come he penetrates my vagina with his penis to continue my pleasure until he reaches orgasm. It was fun to write all this down after many years of practice.

When my partner entered me, he said, "I know that ladies have to help themselves along, so I'll just wait until you do what you have to do. Let me know when to join in." These words were so liberating that he didn't have to wait long! It was really nice to meet a man who was more concerned that I *have* an orgasm than he was with taking credit for having given me one.

———

During my relationship of fourteen years, I climaxed every time using the following position: Missionary-style, woman on her back, man on top, but the woman crosses her legs, forcing the man's penis higher up against her clitoris and also producing increased simulating pressure from the crossed legs.

———

Play with positions. Massage your clit during intercourse. It is a very rare occasion when I come without direct stimulation to my clit. Don't be shy about this; men find it very erotic. You on the couch, him on his knees. Spooning. You on top, front or backward (he can play with your ass this way). Play, play, play.

———

Have you tried using a vibrator in conjunction with having intercourse? Many women have trouble reaching an orgasm in intercourse alone but become multi-orgasmic using a vibrator around the clitoris while having intercourse. The best position is entry from behind, which allows you to stimulate her clitoris as well as use the vibrator. Some feel a vibrator is too mechanical, but for many it is a ticket into orbit.

Ejaculation

Yes, Virginia, and other women and their partners, ejaculation does exist, and, no, it does not seem to be "only" vaginal lubrication nor urine, although traces of both have been found in the fluid that some women expel during orgasmic contractions.

Female ejaculation is possible and occurs in some women. It is an exact carryover of the male one, sans sperm, and more watery. They even produce it by glands that are of the same origin as the males but without the prostatic additions. Actually ejaculation and orgasm is related to the same in males and seems to be a biological innovation for human females, as few other species females experience it.

———

I will speak for me only. It begins with a very strong orgasm that pulsates and squeezes, and then there is a squirting sensation. It is not urine but it has the warm feeling and consistency of urine and is clear. The volume depends on the intensity of the orgasm. If my man teases me long enough, I will squirt very hard the first time. Medical literature I have read says that it secretes from a gland near the vagina. It always feels to me that it is coming from deep inside and squirts out of my vagina.

———

When I use my vibrator alone, I am able to really let myself go. No one to watch and no one to please but me. I do experience that gushing sensation and actually watch myself in the mirror ... but ... but ... I do think at first it *is* urine so I won't do that with a man around. When I do let go, what follows is a clear, highly viscous fluid that pours slowly out of me. It even has an odor like urine, but it is clear and not yellow-tinged. I don't care at all when I am alone. I love the sensations.

———

The first time this happened, I panicked, but realized it was not piss. Just surprised. Now, when she is orgasming I tell her to push, and she floods my mouth with juices. *Wonderful!*

———

I've ejaculated many times from clitoral stimulation alone, which supports my belief that the G-spot is just an anatomical structure, not some special, mystical orgasm button. An orgasm is an orgasm.

———

I remember when I first had a gushing liquid orgasm ... so intense, so good. It was wonderful! After this incredible feeling, I began to think that maybe I had peed. My hubby said no, it didn't taste like that.

I tasted it and it didn't. And the way I felt was so quivery and sensational. I researched it and learned that I am a normal woman! It is absolutely the ultimate feeling!

———

One time, a lady friend and I decided to watch each other masturbate. She was on one side of the bed and I was on the other. She warmed herself up with her fingers, then switched to a vibrator. I lay there watching her, slowly stroking my cock through my panties (Yes, you read that right! I love wearing lingerie!). She worked the vibrator in and out of her vagina for a while as her pleasure built, and soon my cock was bulging against my panties. I could tell she was getting close to orgasm, and she pulled the vibrator out and placed the tip right on her clit, working it in small circles around her most sensitive area, bringing herself to orgasm. As she peaked, her juices sprayed all over the bed. The spraying came in spurts, like a male ejaculation, but was more dispersed. When it was over, she expressed surprise at what happened, saying she had never done that before.

Menopause

If one conceives of menopause as very similar to puberty, a time of wide-ranging body changes that are mainly but not exclusively hormonal, the whole process may not seem as scary nor as mysterious. When their ovaries stop functioning, many women do lose their sex drive. For them, libido is strongly tied to hormone production. Most menopausal women have to face their aging bodies and "invisibility" in a world where youth is all. The lessening desire of many women of this age has to do with shame and anger and the changes in their bodies. Last of all are partner issues: "I've been with ol' Herman for all these years. It's always the same in and out. I'll use menopause as an excuse to stop this stuff once and for all." On the other hand, some women who have been afraid of getting pregnant can now let loose and really enjoy themselves. Women, as you know, are marvelously varied.

I think some women come into their own psychologically and emotionally after age fifty, and this makes them sexually freer. They may reach a peak in their careers, feel less tied to domesticity, have more self-confidence, feel more independent, more aggressive, less vulnerable, especially with men who are fifty-plus, who are becoming more mellow, less vigorous, more sentimental, less intimidating. There's a new equality that is sexually liberating for women. This seems so among my friends.

———

My wife had to have a hysterectomy when she was relatively young, and for a long time that seemed to dampen her libido. As she has gotten older however, it has returned strongly, and she really enjoys lovemaking once again. Patience and understanding are helpful.

———

The symptoms that I thought I was having for the last ten years have all been "cured" by therapy! I am still perimenopausal, and I don't expect to have any more problems. I am experiencing perimenopausal zest, I guess!

———

My wife had to have a hysterectomy last year at age thirty. This is equivalent to surgical menopause, since she lost the uterus as well as both ovaries. The best thing to do is explore a good hormone replacement therapy. My wife tried several, but most only replace estrogen. There are three hormones lost at menopause—estrogen, progesterone, and testosterone. The loss of testosterone leads to the diminished sex drive. Make sure your wife asks about replacing these. Estratest is a brand that contains all three. When my wife started taking testosterone, her sex drive really perked up! Unfortunately, this has subsided recently. We think she may need a stronger dose.

Make sure you demand help from a physician or alternate care provider. If you see an OB/GYN, which was where I received the best results, *insist* on hormone replacement *early*. I spent most of my peri-menopausal and menopausal period caring for an aging mother who had a broken hip. I was so determined not to ever suffer from osteo-porosis that I demanded, and got, HRT. Within six hours of slapping on the first patch, I felt better. When I mentioned this to a physician, he said that the "acid test" for whether or not a woman requires hormone or other therapy is how she feels after she has begun it. Even though I was only perimenopausal, for the first time I got pushy with my OB/GYN, and got relief. It can be absolute hell, it really can. Other friends have gone the herb and meditation route with equal success, but it didn't work for me. Please make sure you pay more attention than ever to your physical and mental well-being. On a very cheery note, sex becomes much, much better ... with the right man. Menopause and post-menopause is definitely the best part of life.

What I resented when I first began making inquiries of my doctors is that all the printed information they had was from drug companies. Women have to inform themselves on the issues, and it's pretty con-fusing. I suspect that many of the symptoms that are attributed to per-imenopause are really not directly related to it, but are related to other things happening in a woman's life at the time she may be going through perimenopause. Depression happens for a variety of reasons; so does anxiety. Symptom relief can be had by good diet, exercise, and stress reduction, but that is easier said than done.

It is fairly common for a woman to suffer a great loss of libido after menopause. If your doctor is unwilling to explore options with you, it's time to find another doctor. There has been success in restoring the libido with testosterone patches for post-menopausal women. Look for a doctor who is up to date with the current treatments and who is willing to take your problem seriously.

———

I am in my mid-fifties, and my wife and I have lived through her menopause and come out fine, perhaps better for it. She never totally lost her *interest* in sex, but clearly, for a while, she did not *enjoy* it. She made sure that I got sex in one form or another, but if *she* didn't enjoy it, it was difficult for *me* to enjoy it. Then a great thing happened. A lifelong friend of hers, who had gone through menopause a year earlier, told my wife how she had solved the problem. On the friend's advice my wife went to Planned Parenthood, where they gave her a thorough exam and then gave her a year's prescription for estrogen pills. Bang! In a few days she was her old self again, only more so. It has been five or six years since that time, and we fuck like rabbits all the time. Without question, she *enjoys* it. And so do I.

———

I'm a guy, so I don't know much of the feminine mindset regarding this issue. I must say that as I've entered my forties, my own mortality has become all the more obvious. I have sensed the need in my life for more positive affirmation by those I love, and I'm not undergoing "menopause" . . . maybe a bit of "midlife." I said all that to say this: Beyond the doctors, hormones, herbs, I encourage you to affirm your wife's desirability and become all the more verbal about your love for her and your attraction to her. If you've never or ever done it before, express how important she is to you; don't assume she knows just because it's apparent to you. Go out of your way to wine and dine her. Sit down together and consider the positives that come with age. My wife and I are free to date again as our children are old enough to care for themselves. Maybe you can do more traveling or perhaps just surprise her by packing an overnight bag for both of you and sweeping her away to dinner and a nice hotel you've never been to. (P.S.: Don't forget her make-up!). Seek creative ways to express your love and interest, ways to encourage and affirm her, and I believe you'll never regret it. There is nothing that turns my wife on faster than to feel accepted and cherished. When we as husbands do things that show our appreciation of our spouses, it makes them feel a bit more special. Who knows what kind of miracles a tangible demonstration of affection and love might do for any of our wives.

———

As I've had children, gotten older, started menopause, my moistness has changed. I'd like to offer my deepest most heartfelt thanks for the inventor of water-based lubricants! I use lubes for masturbating and for sex. Warmed lube is very nice.

CHAPTER 14

Relationship
Middles and Endings

Even the most solitary of humans has relationships, even if it's merely a nodding acquaintance with the person who delivers the mail. When most of us use the word relationship. however, it's shorthand for an intimate relationship, a sexual relationship, or both—sort of Relationship with a capital R. Sex can take place within the context of an intimate relationship or not, and within various other kinds of relationships. We all know relationships that take place without any sex too, but most of us are happier when we successfully combine the two.

Keeping the Spark Alive

Do the initial delicious throes of passion necessarily have to fade into everyday humdrum? Does the person whose very presence once set your heart beating wildly have to dwindle into just old Whoosis who steals the covers? How to keep sexual sparkle in long-term relationships is a subject of vital interest.

Focus on the fun things in your relationship and the sex should follow naturally. Go for hikes, picnics, ice skating, amusement parks, a ball game, ice cream, a boat ride ... anything where you can enjoy each other's company and rekindle the reasons you fell in love.

———

Spontaneity has its place and I adore it, but I also like really planning for sex well in advance. I have a busy life, and I tend to be attracted to women who are also busy, so finding time to get together can be problematic. I've noticed that when I have a specific date for sex on my calendar, maybe arranged weeks and weeks ahead, it tends to build my anticipation and subsequent enjoyment a great deal. I'm thinking about it for a while, thinking of things I'd like to have happen, playing it over in my mind. When I first heard a relationship expert say, "If you want to have good sex put it on your calendar," I thought it was a joke. In practice it turns out to be a brilliant suggestion. Grabbing a burger at McDonald's is quick and easy and spontaneous. Having a fine meal at the Four Seasons requires some forethought. There's a place for each in a well-rounded relationship. Margo Anand refers to these extremes as "gourmet sex" and "fast food sex," and says that even she, a Tantra master, likes some of each.

———

Lovemaking is more an act of *giving* than one of *receiving*. Sure, it can be highly satisfying if both of you are horny, but it can still be mutually satisfying if only one of you is, if you approach it with the right attitude. In a few weeks I will have been married to the same woman for thirty-five years. We will have been having sex for nearly forty years. Without any doubt, one reason why we have stayed together for so long is that we don't require that both partners have to be fiercely horny at the same moment. Throughout the years my sexual needs have been about twice as frequent as hers. Rarely (maybe never) has she failed to enjoy the opportunity to get me off with a blow job or a hand job, anal sex, or intercourse. Often the act of doing me was enough to get her horny too. So then I would pitch in and help to get her off. Less commonly, she wants it and I don't. So I'm "on hand" for her (and that usually gets me horny too). I generally try to let her initiate sex, so that I don't wear the woman out. We know each other well enough that we can figure out each other's wants. We enjoy sex. The giving attitude that we share heightens the enjoyment. It doesn't matter how often you are horny (within reason, of course). What matters is your attitude toward your partner's desires. If you can find pleasure in satisfying him, he will be happy with you, I'm sure.

————

There are definite benefits to planned sex. The hours leading up to it can be filled with flirting and foreplay, which can often be as nice as the main event.

————

It's tough early on with the young ones, but it gets better. We make appointments for sex now. Spontaneity is for wiping noses.

————

My husband and I have three children. We both have jobs and we participate in youth activities. When we tried to have sex during the middle of the night, when we awakened in the morning, or on Saturday afternoons, inevitably there would be an interruption. Our lives have not become any less hectic, but I am happy to say we have solved the problem. Right after our children go to sleep at night they sleep soundly and don't need us. Initially once a week, but now a least three times a week, once the children have gone to sleep is our time alone—no TV, work, or anything else. We usually give each other massages with baby oil. We have time to talk, and the massages relieve stress and make our bodies wonderfully soft to the touch. When we are tired we just fall asleep embracing each other's naked bodies. Other times we have wonderful sex. Every time is a peaceful, uninterrupted moment of intimacy.

———

When two people come together they form a third entity greater than themselves—a relationship. Each relationship has its own natural rhythm, its own intimate dance, like breathing. In the influx stage you feel deeply connected to the other and the union of your love fills you with gladness. Then there will be other times when you feel that all that was in your grasp is moving away from you, or you from it. At these times we often feel disconnected. If we don't understand the process, we may begin to doubt ourselves and our partners. Sometimes we retreat, feeling like they don't love us in the same way. These doubts can begin to erode the link that still binds us. Each relationship phase has a distinct purpose. The outward phase allows us to go forth into the world, to learn more about ourselves, and to grow in new ways. The inward phase allows us to return once more to the warm hearth as stronger, wiser people who are more aware of the purpose of our love and lives. To stay connected during the expiration phase of a relationship, you need to keep faith in the love that initially brought you together. Reenacting simple rituals and gestures of courtship, such as writing love letters or doing something thoughtful, can help foster that good will between you. Given time, the relationship will shift in direction and draw itself inward once more. So it goes through the lifetime of each relationship.

———

Men, if you remember they are your children also and do your part in caring for them, and show her that you care for her, sex will be there—probably more sex than you can handle.

———

The dearly beloved and I had a bit of a quandary on our hands this evening. He was horny, I was horny, but I was also in the midst of cooking dinner and he had to catch a bus to work in less than twenty-five minutes. Yet somehow we managed to produce two orgasms (one each) without the kids ever noticing we were gone, still get supper on the table with time to have his belly properly fed, *and* he caught his bus on time. What's more, I don't think I've ever had an orgasm quite as intense. Normally, I prefer the long drawn-out style of lovemaking, but I've got to admit haste has its place.

Get healthy together. Walk every evening for fifteen or twenty minutes. Eat foods that don't sap your energy in the evenings. Go out of the way to touch each other, even if you're sure there will be no sex—kiss, hold hands, cuddle, pat a butt, brush up against her breast, peek at her when she's showering or changing. Give each other a warm physical greeting when you come home after a day of work. (This is actually great for the kids to see two loving adults in physical contact. Kids learn by imitation.) Date each other. Plan intimate evenings and don't break your dates. When our kids were young we had no money to go out or even pay a baby-sitter, so when they were tucked away in bed we would both dress up and have an intimate candlelight dinner, cocktails, or dessert. Sometimes he would even walk out the back door and come in the front door with flowers, as if he were coming over for a visit! Plan mini-vacations. A weekend at a local motel, kids with relatives or friends. For a while we shared kid-sleepover duties with a neighbor so we could have the house to ourselves for an evening. If she likes cunnilingus from time to time give her a "blow job" without expecting anything in return. Lastly, talk with her.

We talk a lot about sex when we can. We watch videos. We talk some more. We try new things. We go new places. We talk about things that sound fun but we would probably never do. We talk about things we would like to do and how we would like to do them.

Husband and I were discussing our current schedule: work, eat, sleep, work, eat, sleep, and how to set it up so that we could insert more sex into the sequence. We talked about eating dinner too late and that sex after that is somehow less than fun, but then, we work late and we still need to eat. We talked about being too tired, another byproduct of work and eating (gotta cook). I volunteered that often, although I may seem quite tired, some TLC like a back rub that becomes something else could get my adrenaline going again. He looked at me with a gleam in his eye and asked, "Really?" We have been married for fifteen years. Enough cannot be said for loving communication. If you aren't communicating with the person you love, you are cheating both parties. Jeez, he really *can't* read my mind!

———

This is in response to the gay man who is feeling depressed by the amount and by the "efficient and mechanical" nature of the sex he has with his partner of twenty-two years. I am no New Age positive thinker, but there is something to be said about looking at the glass as half-full. What if he were sick or injured or could not have sex? What if his partner were a chronic liar or a spendthrift? The bad "what if's" are infinite, but there is a solid relationship here that is not destructive. They do not fight or argue, and there is respect in the relationship. Many would love to have had successful careers and be financially secure. It just isn't productive to look back over twenty-two years and yearn for a lost youth. By his own words, sexual adventures were not his desire. Often we make our own cage and then get in it. We must take responsibility for our choices and not blame the consequences on others. If his partner is colder than he prefers, perhaps he could have friends (some friendships are better than sex), take a hobby, even a pet. It seems unlikely that he or his friend will change their sexual habits at this late date. Rather than starting over with someone new, it is possible for him to alter his feelings by taking a wider view, giving more weight to the good things, changing activities, and altering expectations. The perfect marriage is hard to come by, but we can decide to be happy, to love, and to make adjustments.

Libido

A lack of sexual desire is the singular most frequent complaint marriage counselors and sex therapists hear about today. Sometimes the cause(s) are physical—ill health, stress, hormonal changes; sometimes they are psychological—depression, anxiety, unaddressed relationship problems. Often the causes are varied. In any case, there is always something that can be done to make the situation better, if not necessarily ideal, if both partners are willing to go exploring.

My wife went through a period when she didn't care if we had sex or not, and when we did, she was just going through the motions. She had been multi-orgasmic while we were dating and up until the birth of our second child. After our daughter was born, though, she lost interest and never climaxed. She was diagnosed with clinical depression. Along with a lack of interest in sex, she also began to lack patience with me and the kids, and began not caring about her personal appearance. Once she started taking medication for it, things improved. We still don't have sex as often as I'd like, but she will initiate it on occasion and will have an occasional multiple orgasm. The other items associated with her depression also changed. By the way, I also do the majority of the housework. Even though my wife didn't want sex, she told me she still wanted me and needed me. It can be fixed, but you may need medical attention.

———

Another reason why women want sex less often than men is because they suffer from the orgasm gap. Only 29 percent of women are coming on a regular basis (compared to 75 percent of men) in sex. No wonder women are less interested. Women's low orgasm rate (imagine only a third of men having regular orgasms) is not due to socialization alone but to the definition of sex as primarily intercourse that gives men direct stimulation but does not stimulate most women's clitoris enough to have orgasms. What women (and men who want more enthusiastic partners) need is a new definition of sex that includes manual and oral sex to orgasm. The orgasm gap and its causes and solutions are discussed in the book, *Are We Having Fun Yet?*

It is OK for a woman to want sex? It is OK to crave it, need it, want it so badly that you can hardly stand it? Women need to reclaim their sexuality. Your sexuality is a part of who you are. It is more than just the miracle of making a human life, and it is more than sharing an intense orgasm with a partner. And it can be just as magical with a person that you don't know as with a person you've known for years.

I get frustrated with the hormonal effects of long-term nursing. I expect they are quite intentional (from Nature's point of view), but they sure can be a nuisance. What has worked for me in the past, and extremely well, was increasing the amount of exercise I do, dramatically. Exercise that builds muscle also increases the amount of testosterone in a woman's body, which is the major hormone associated with libido in both genders. I know lots of women quake at the thought of lifting weights, but it does build muscle. And it firms areas that childbearing has a tendency to soften, a very nice side effect. It sounds simplistic, that exercise would alter body chemistry to such a degree, but it works.

I checked a book out of the public library quite a while ago. It was all about the effects of hormones on sexual desire. It was fascinating reading, and one of the most handy features was a chart for each hormone: what effect it has, factors to increase or decrease it naturally, and so on. I do recall weight-lifting being mentioned as a means to influence testosterone, especially in women.

A thirty-two-year-old female complained that her fifty-two-year-old husband had no desire for sex and that he always had a cold. I agree that there is probably more to his lack of sexual desire than his cold, and I also think there is a possibility that the cold and the lack of sexual desire might have a common cause—diet. The average American often eats combinations of foods that do not digest well together. This inefficient digestion drains energy from the body and can cause it to be more susceptible to disease. There are a number of books available on the subject of proper food combining.

The guy who complacently says men are more interested in sex is dead wrong, in my opinion. For most men, sex is a tool, if you'll forgive the expression, used to gain power or dominance. Any Don Juan will tell you that the thrill is in the chase, not the actual sex. I think most women are far more interested in sex for its own sake. They can dally at it for hours, while men race ahead to the orgasm and then go to sleep. If you doubt that sex is a power thing for men, check out our obsession with penis size, which has more to do with psyching out other men than with women's enjoyment. Male gorillas fighting to dominate get erections.

Here is an option for the woman with touch deprivation: get a dog or cat. While a pet won't satisfy her sexual needs (one would hope), it is very therapeutic to pet and cuddle. Having a loyal, loving, four-legged friend helps to combat loneliness. It has been medically proven that petting an animal lowers one's heart rate and can help control stress. Also, taking a dog on walks or to the park may help with meeting people. A pooch can be an excellent icebreaker.

To the man who patronizingly wondered if women are not as sexually turned on as men, my answer is that men are trained to be more obviously turned on. There aren't many clubs for women (Shlongs instead of Hooters), nor men who show their cocks in movies. If women had more access in the general media to stuff that would turn them on, maybe things would be different. As it stands, women get Sean Connery with women half his age in movies and Dennis Franz's butt on television instead of David Duchovny's. Even though our society tells women what sluts they are for wanting to see naked men, and women are raped, incested against, have to deal with periods, births, and ageism, they are still interested in sex ... which, I think, makes them more interested in sex than men.

Meds and Drugs

Anything that is ingested (eaten, smoked, injected, inserted) that has a physical effect upon the body will undoubtedly have other effects that were not part of the original purpose. Why, then, are so many people surprised when anything from alcohol to antidepressants create profound changes in sexual functioning—whether it be desire, arousal, or orgasmic capacity? There are many new drugs on the market, and each person's body chemistry varies in its reactions to them. If there is a medicine that you need to take that cramps your sexual style, keep working with your physician until some livable arrangement can be found.

Years back I was taking Zoloft and Paxil, both prescription selective serotonin reuptake inhibitors (a.k.a., mind-altering drugs). While they had no effect on my depression, they had an effect on my dick. Once aroused, I could stay hard indefinitely but never ejaculate. At first it was kind of fun. After two hours the novelty starts wearing off. After four hours I was mightily frustrated, and both of us were sore and exhausted. The lack of sleep messed up our daytime lives too, and I abandoned the drugs after a few weeks. If she's wondering why he doesn't come, I imagine that taking antidepressants is something a guy might not talk about freely. There's an awfully big stigma surrounding mental health care.

———

More than twenty years ago I got some yohimbe from an herbalist and made tea with it. Yohimbe made me extremely euphoric and potent. I got a horrible hangover from it, including a backache afterward. I was warned not to drink alcohol with yohimbe as it would play hell with my blood pressure. Doctors prescribe yohimbe for impotence. Talk to your doctor before you go to an herbalist.

———

After months of taking those herbal performance enhancers to no noticeable effect, I stopped as of last week. Since then I've felt the horniest I can remember. Last night after ejaculating I remained hard for several minutes. I've been masturbating more than ever.

———

Yohimbe works well; I use the scrip from my M.D. Green oats and nettles from Puritans's Pride seem to help too. Introital does a fair job also. Get in shape, work out, exercise. And, if you can, stop aging.

———

I used to take DHEA regularly and it made me hornier than a three-peckered goat! I finally decided to quit taking it because the wife couldn't keep up. By the way, she took it too for a while and it helped her drive. Now I'm wishing she was still taking it. It may or may not work for you, and your mileage may vary.

———

I was on an antidepressant known as Manerix (trade name moclobemide) for about a year. Initially my libido was limited (likely as a result of the depression), but once that lifted, my libido balanced out. Manerix doesn't seem to inhibit desire, and there is even some evidence that it may enhance it.

———

After taking Prozac for several years, I began having trouble reaching orgasm. My doctor had me try the others, but the side effects were bad for me. Finally I began taking Wellbutrin. I don't think this drug is as "clean" in helping with the depression; however, it does not effect my ability to achieve orgasm.

I am on Paxil and have been for about a year now. I lost my libido due to depression, started on Paxil, and lost even more of my sex drive. Paxil seems to work pretty well for depression and, so far the only side effects have been loss of libido (huge) and difficulty achieving orgasms. I can literally go for hours without having an orgasm. Like they say, be careful what you ask for!

I'm on Prozac. It's made me mildly less horny. The real problem is that it's much harder for me to come now. I used to be able to come pretty effortlessly, now I've got to both work and pray, and it's still pretty hit or miss. What I did about it: I bought a vibrator (a godsend), and I tell my partners that I'm a tough nut to crack, tell them why, and give them lots of feedback. I tell them that it still feels great even if I don't come (assuming that is the case, which it unfortunately is in most cases).

I was taking Zoloft for about four years. A side effect for me was increased libido but inability to orgasm. I went crazy. It was horrible. This summer I changed to Luvox, and my libido has dropped by 50 percent. I don't like that, but at least now I *can* orgasm.

I took Zoloft for a while and noticed a complete downturn in my horniness. But when I started feeling better, I stopped taking it, and *zoom!* My libido shot up to the stratosphere, its normal level. How did I start feeling better again? By running. The doc said that when you exercise regularly, you create your own antidepressants.

When It's Over

We've spoken here of finding relationships, maintaining relationships, and improving relationships. Sometimes, no matter how hard someone has tried, it becomes necessary to end a relationship. And, while all endings have an element of sadness to them, especially in cases where love or lust or even respect has disappeared, this stage of the process can be done with style, grace, and a minimum of damage to the parties involved when someone is willing to make that effort.

I had a man break up with me in a two-minute phone conversation. We'd last slept together a week before that. Speaking slowly and insistently, as if to a child, he said it wasn't working out between us, but that I'd done nothing about which I needed to be ashamed. He made it quite clear that he wanted nothing more to do with me for the time being, "but would probably be back in touch someday." Whether we're talking about the passive avoidance of a lover one wants to be rid of or the kind of hit-and-run I experienced, the cowardly refusal of one partner to allow for unhurried and caring discussion at the end of a sexual involvement is a violation of the other, like a rape.

———

I have a friend who broke up with a series of boyfriends, and she always complained bitterly when she felt that they had not handled the break-ups in a satisfactory way. But I always wondered when she complained, "What is a satisfactory way?" Are people supposed to call and say, "I'm just calling because I don't want to speak to you!" There may be a tendency to list reasons for the break-up; this could be pointlessly hurtful. I also don't believe that people learn from break-ups very much that is transferable to other relationships. The only thing I learned was that I didn't get along very well with that particular person, and that break-ups were painful, awkward, and somewhat embarrassing.

———

Two of the women I dated both had extreme sales personalities. So while on the inside they were probably trying to figure out what they thought of me and whether they wanted to continue seeing me or not, on the outside the message they were giving me was "Yes, yes, yes—I like you, I like you, I like you." The transition from that message to not even returning a phone call is certainly abrupt and disconcerting. In addition, recently a woman said to me on the phone (we'd only gone out once), "Well, this was nice. I'm glad you called. So, you should call me again, or I'll call you sometime." Yet her meaning—which in some subtle way I picked up from her tone—was the exact opposite of her words. Her meaning was (or seemed to be): "This is over. Please don't call me again—I certainly won't be calling you."

———

A woman I've recently dated a little complained to me that men (and she's gone out with a lot of men in the past couple of years, though usually only once or twice with each of them) often talk prematurely (in her view) about things they're going to do together in the future, as if it were all a done deal. So I'm trying to be conscious not to do that. At the same time, it only seems natural to discuss, for example, movies that are coming out soon that we both might like to see. I guess the idea here is not to get too far ahead of ourselves.

———

For the people who want to get on with their lives after a relationship has ended, running a witty ad will get you a lot of attention, but please keep in mind that the blind leading the blind tend to walk into traffic! Give yourself time after a relationship ends.

———

Take heart, it does get better. You don't ever want to lose the memories of the good times, but at the same time you need to remember and temper them with the reason(s) that forced you into making the decision. You know in your heart that it was the right thing to do. The trick is to remember that when you start having those second thoughts, those ones that come during the loneliest times, and you start wondering if it was really that bad. Don't give in to those. You did what you had to do to protect yourself emotionally. Remember that *no one* is going to take care of you better than yourself, especially when the decisions are the hardest to make.

I have been dumped by too many of those "sensitive caring men" (from sophisticated city types to those from the cornfields of Nebraska) to honestly believe it! *Dumped* is my term, by the way, probably not theirs, because they just cut off all contact, no big fight, nothing to indicate why. To me that is *the* most adolescent way to communicate your desire to end the thing. *Just say something,* then maybe I'd see you as a rational adult, Mr.-Caring -Sensitive-Guy.

It's good to end things in person. Break-up phone calls are hell: painful and expensive. Plus, when you break up in person you can have "break-up sex," which is, arguably, better than the much-vaunted "make-up sex."

To the people who are stopping strangers on the street asking them if they heard about your divorce: Please know that you will get through this. You will tell fewer and fewer people, and before you know it only a select group or few will be your support.

For you who are out of a relationship that has lasted three or four years, let me give you my point of view:

1. I've never been a better person.
2. I've never been a better father.
3. I've never felt this kind of happiness before.
4. I'm still working on me. . . .
5. Yes there is still some pain, but I still remember the love and great times of a long-term relationship!

Postscript

Some people may find that ending a book of sex tips with a section on the end of relationships is depressing. If so, you could, of course, quickly riffle the pages back to chapter 1, The Single State, for uplifting and forward-thinking reading. To save you the trouble, I will end instead with several comments on the pleasures of living alone that might have been included in that chapter but follow here instead.

Some suggestions to stave off loneliness: If you like animals (and your apartment allows them), get a pet. Walking a dog gives you a reason to get out and gives people an opening to talk to you. Pets are really good company, too. Make a list of books that you always wanted to read, and go for it. Take up a new hobby. Join a club or organization that interests you. It's a great way to meet people, and you have a similar interest to talk about from the start. Have a regular night to invite friends over. Center it around dinner, a TV show, gab fest. Volunteer work is fulfilling and another opportunity to meet new people. Pick a topic to research on the Net (I love to do this, but you may be thinking *yick*). Search out games to play on the Net. There are lots of great games out there, both interactive and not.

———

I am alone the majority of the time that I am at home. There are times that I get lonely or bored, but then there are the rest of the times when I'm thrilled to be by myself. I hang out with my cats, watch TV, do some crafts, play on the computer, have sex when I'm lucky enough to get some. The best part of having your own place is being able to live by your own rules and do what you want there. I hardly ever wear a stitch of clothing when I'm home. As soon as I get in the door, the clothes go flying. I really like living by myself. If you get lonely, have some friends or family over or visit them at their place.

———

You can wander around totally naked. You can dance wildly. You don't have to do the dishes until *you* are ready to do them or run out of clean ones, whichever comes first.

———

You can masturbate in the kitchen. If you really need someone there, you could get a Betta fish. The idea is to have just enough friends that you feel a nice balance between company and alone. A nice balance keeps things looking bright!

Index

A

Allen, Woody, 84
allergy to latex, 74, 76, 80–1, 113, 193
American Social Health Association, 81
anal masturbation, 84, 90, 94
anal sex, 118, 122, 200, 204
   and communication and lubrication, 4, 80, 153, 156
   and condoms/cleanliness, 151, 154, 158
   and fisting, 167–9
   play, 82, 99–100, 133, 137, 140, 143, 149–60
   and vaginal intercourse, 82, 151, 154
Anand, Margot, 193, 216
anatomy
   men's, 178–87
   women's, 198–201
anilingus, 152, 154, 156
Antoniou, Laura, 173
arginine, 81
arousal, 126, 201–3, 214
   men and women, 98–9, 104–5
"Ask Isadora," 1–2, 88
ass (*see also* anal sex), 98, 101–2
Astroglide (*see also* lubrication), 90, 152, 154, 169
attractiveness (*see also* turn-ons), 7, 9, 36, 64
autofellatio, 93

B

balls (*see also* oral sex on a man; sex play), 90, 136, 140, 146
   shaving, 71
B&D, 171–6
benzocaine, 153
birth control (*see also* condoms), 68, 74–8, 163, 202
bisexuality (*see also* polyamory; threesomes), 53
blow jobs (*see also* oral sex on a man), 99–100
   on one's self, 93–5
body (*see also* specific parts of the body; attractiveness), 63–82
   comfort with one's own, 64–5
   tastes, 65–7
   smells, 67–8
   hair, 68–73
body hair, 68–73
body image, 63–5, 85
books recommended, 78, 118–9, 152, 173, 174, 193, 202, 222

"bottoming," 151, 172

breasts, 31, 101–2, 103, 107–10

and underside crease, 101–2, 107

brushes, 98, 100–1, 103

butt plugs (*see also* toys), 150, 155, 159

C

cervix, 168–69

Chia and Arana, 193

circumcision, 89, 185–7

cleanliness

and washing, 136, 138

and anal play, 151, 154, 158

clitoral and/or G-spot stimulation (*see also* clitoris; intercourse; oral sex on a woman; orgasm; sex play), 87, 105–6, 122, 198–201, 209

clitoris, 100, 101, 120–2, 127–9, 198–203

Comfort, Alex, 161

coming (*see also* orgasm), 102–3

communication, 12, 17, 18, 23, 25, 37, 47–8

communication about sex, 41–2, 54, 74, 102, 207, 219–20

and anal sex, 4, 80, 153, 156

and dating, 23, 25, 31

and fisting, 167

and relationship, 48

threesomes, 163–5

condoms, 74–8, 117, 123, 176

and anal sex, 151, 154

brands and qualities, 74–8, 117

and breaking, 76–7

and latex allergies, 74, 76,

80–81, 113, 193

and threesomes, 163–4

coupling, 45–61

"creative sex play," 161–76

cross-dressing, 165–7

cultural convention, 33, 55, 83, 85, 86

and gender roles, 13–5, 31, 38

cum, 66–7, 108, 194–6

cunnilingus (*see also* oral sex on a woman), 117, 203, 219

D

D&S, 171–2

dating, 23–44

friends and lovers, 33–5, 41

"I'll call you," 37–41

nice guys, 35–37

paying the bill, 31–2

and sex, 14, 41–4

as shopping, 24–7

turn-offs, 31–3

turn-ons, 27–30

decision making, 48, 49

Depo-Provera, 78

depression, 221, 224–6

DHEA, 225

diabetes, 187

diet, 223

and genital herpes, 81

and taste of semen, 66–7

dildo (*see also* toys), 60

doggie-style, 102, 118, 122–3, 167

Don Juan, 223

E

ears, 100

Easton and Liszt, 174

ejaculation
early, 119, 120
female, 123, 198, 208–10
and orgasm, 192–6
Encore, Inc., 187
endorphins, 104, 172
enemas, 154, 158–60
erections, 187–91
resources, 187
exercise, 222, 225, 226
PC muscles, 158, 205–6
eye contact (*see also* face), 30, 119, 139, 194

F

face (*see also* eye contact), 102, 106, 116, 118
"facials," 195
fellatio (*see also* oral sex on a man), 76, 103, 157
fisting, 167–9
Five Freedoms, 46
flavor enhancers (*see also* taste), 138
ForPlay lube (*see also* lubrication), 79
foreplay (*see also* sex play), 41–2, 97–114, 133, 200
frenulum, 91
friends and lovers, 33–5, 41, 51

G

gay male subculture, 181–2
genital herpes, 81–2
genital warts, 81
group sex, 165
G-spot (*see also* clitoral and/or G-

spot stimulation) 120, 159, 176, 198–201

H

hair, on head (*see also* body hair), 103, 139
hand balling. *See* fisting
hand jobs (*see also* sex play), 99–100, 106, 139–40
Haydon, Laura, 118–19
Hepatitis C, 73, 80
herbal performance enhancers, 225
HIV, 73, 80, 151
hormones, 200, 202, 203, 210, 211–2, 222
and menstruation, 74
post-orgasm, 89
replacement, 211–3
and touch, 104
hydrocele, 184
hysterectomy, 211

I

"I'll call you," 24, 37–41
Impotence Institute of America, 187
intercourse (*see also* condoms; sex play), 97, 104, 105, 115–24, 208
and climaxing, 86, 206
defined, 97, 115, 221
Internet (*see also* Web site resources), 16–8, 164, 183
Internet/personal ad relationships, 7, 16–8, 51, 163
and meeting, 17–8, 25, 50

J

jealousy, 53, 54, 163
jelquing, 182, 183
Joy of Sex, The, 161

K

Kama Sutra, 205
Kegel exercises, 168
kissing (*see also* oral sex; intercourse; sex play), 30, 44, 106, 131
    first kisses, 26, 27, 42–43

L

latex, 74, 76, 80–1, 113, 193
lesbians, 13–4, 19, 120–1
libido, 78, 210–3, 221–6
    differing between partners,
      213–4, 223
    and meds, drugs, 224–6
loneliness, 8, 10, 231–2
love, 48
    and sex, 48, 51
lovemaking, 98, 99, 100, 155
    as giving, 216–7
lubrication, 79–80, 120, 214
    and anal play, 4, 80, 152, 154,
      156, 157
    and condoms, 75–6
    and fisting, 167–8
    glycerin-based, 79, 81
    and masturbating, 89–9, 96
    and numbing, 79
    water-based, 167, 214
lysine, 81

M

magazines, 69, 88–9

Manerix, 225
Mardi Gras, 170
marriage, 21, 47, 52–7
massage, 7, 101
masturbation, 83–6
    anal, 84
    men, 88–93, 95
    oral, 93–5
    with a partner, 86, 94–6, 195,
      202, 210
    women, 84–8, 205, 206
meds and drugs, 224–6
meeting, 11–9
men, 177–96
menopause, 202, 205, 210–4
menstruation, 73–4, 77–8
    cramps, 74, 85–6
mirrors, 85, 100, 118, 169, 209
monogamy, 52–7
Morin, Jack, 152
morning-after pill, 77

N

Nair, 70–71
natural family planning, 78
necks, 103, 107, 109, 127
"nice," 49–51
"nice guys," 35–7
nipples, 3, 30
    and breasts, 107–10
    hair, 69, 70
    nursing, 222

O

oral sex, 103
    on a woman, 70, 72, 73, 75,
      125–34
      and penetration, 127, 130

on a man, 71, 76, 135–47, 196
    deep throating, 140, 142
    swallowing, 65–7, 140,
      142, 144
    taste of semen, 65–7
orgasm (*see also* anal play;
  erections; intercourse; oral sex;
  sex play) 219
    and ejaculating, 192–6
    gap, women's and men's,
      221–2
    and masturbation, 85–94
    and meds, drugs, 224–6
    multiple, 91, 92, 120, 190, 192,
      200
    partner's, 102
    women, 201–10
Osbon Medical Systems, 187
OVA, 169

P

Paxil, 224, 226
PC muscle, 205–6
pearl necklace, 107–8
penis (*see also* anal play; intercourse; masturbation; oral sex;
  sex play), 136, 143, 178–87
    connected to nips, 107
    pleasure areas, 122, 143, 144,
     178
    size and shape, 65, 118,
     178–84, 188, 223
perineum, 99, 137, 140
phone sex, 58, 59, 84
physical appearance, 10, 29
    and age, 13
    and height, 13, 14, 122
    and lesbians, 13–4
    and weight, 10, 65

Pill, the, 75, 77–8
Planned Parenthood, 77–8, 213
polyamory, 32, 52–7
positions, 116, 117, 119–23, 142,
  208
    and anal sex, 151, 158
    doggie-style, 102, 118, 122–3,
     167
    and hand jobs, 99, 106
    missionary, 116, 119
    and oral sex, 127, 130, 137,
     144
    woman to woman, 120–1
power play, 171–6
pre-cum, 93, 143, 145
pregnancy (*see also* birth control),
  73, 75, 77, 80, 119, 200
    fear of, 49, 118, 211
privacy, 50–1
prostrate, 99–100, 137, 156, 194
    and perineum, 137, 140
Prozac, 226
pubes, 68–73

Q

QSM, 172, 174

R

rejection, 38–41
relationships, 45–51, 215
    balance in, 47–50
    and children, 217–9
    endings, 40, 227–31
    first sex together, 41–4
    friends and lovers, 11, 17,
     33–5, 41, 51, 53
    historical perspectives, 45, 47,
     52

keeping spark alive, 216–20
long-distance, 17, 57–61
and love, 48
monogamy and polyamory,
    52–7
new, 46–50
nature of, 46–7, 49, 51, 52,
    61, 218
and uncertainty, 49–50
Replens, 203
rimming (*see also* anal play,
  anilingus), 137, 143, 146, 159

S

S&M, 171, 174
Satir, Virginia, 46
scrotum (*see also* balls; testes), 184
    shaving, 71–3
secrecy and privacy, 50–1
semen, 65–7
sex, 99, 100, 115, 155
    first time with someone,
        41–4
    and gender, 15, 25, 26, 27, 37,
        51, 98–9, 223–4
    and love, 48, 49, 51
    and menstruation, 73–4
    planned, 216–9
    as reward, 27, 51
sex play (*see also* anal play; intercourse; oral sex), 97–114
sex talk, 30, 98, 110–2, 138, 143
sexual dysfunction, 202
sexual housekeeping, 123–4
Sexuality Forum, 2–4, 162
shaving, 68–73, 120
shyness, 12
single, being, 5–22, 231–2

and searching for a sweetie,
    11–22
sixty-nine (69), 128, 129, 152, 157,
    196, 207
smells, 67–8, 76, 85, 126, 130
STDs, 75, 80–2, 151, 163
    fear of, 49
stromboli, 94
swinging (*see also* polyamory;
    threesomes), 46, 54, 164

T

Tantric sex, 191, 193, 216
Taoist-based method, 193
tastes (*see also* oral sex), 65–7, 76,
    126, 130–1, 138
testes (*see also* balls), 140
    smell, 67, 130
testosterone, 20, 104, 222
    in women, 211–3, 222
threesomes, 55, 162–5
"topping," 151, 172
touch, 7, 29, 30, 104, 220, 223
toys, 80, 98, 112–4, 150, 156,
    175
turn-offs, 31–3
turn-ons, 27–30

U

urethra, 201
urinary tract infection (UTI), 82,
    151

V

vacuum pumps, 90, 180–1, 187
vagina (*see also* clitoris; G-spot;

intercourse; oral sex; sex play), 126, 183

air from, 117

and anal play/infection, 151, 154

dryness/wetness, 203, 207, 214

frontal wall, 119

smell, 67–8

vaginitis and yeast infections, 79–81, 113, 169

varieties, 161–6

Viagra, 190–1, 202

vibrators (*see also* toys), 112–3, 153, 159, 207–10, 226

voyeurism and exhibitionism, 170–1, 174, 202

W

water drinking, 66

Web site resources, 2, 75, 81, 84, 111, 120, 174, 175, 182, 188, 205

weight lifting, 222

women, 197–214, 222

anatomy, 198–201

words (*see also* sex talk), 89, 135–6

work, relationships at, 20, 34

X

x-rated films, 156, 181, 202

Y

yohimbe, 225

Z

Zoloft, 224, 226

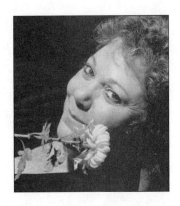

About the Author

Isadora Alman is a California licensed Marriage and Family Therapist and a Board certified sexologist. She was a recently divorced real estate agent back in 1979, when, at the suggestion of a friend, she first took the training for phone line volunteers at San Francisco Sex Information. She enjoyed working with the community of people who supported open discussion of sexuality so much—"dealing with people's sexual and emotional secrets was far more interesting to me than dealing with their financial ones"—that she hung around the organization for more than a dozen years, as phone volunteer, shift supervisor, training staff, outreach liaison, and member of the Board of Directors. Eventually she became credentialed as a psychotherapist and began a small private counseling practice focusing on social skills and sexuality. In 1984 she approached the editor of the *San Francisco Bay Guardian,* the local alternative weekly which had a large personal advertising section, with the idea of a column for the readers and the placers of those ads. The rest is history.

Besides her column, which is currently being carried in sixteen or so weekly papers, she is the author of *Sex Information: May I Help*

You? (originally published as *Aural Sex & Verbal Intercourse* by Down There Press), a fictionalized account of her volunteer time with San Francisco Sex Information, and two collections of questions and answers from her column, *Ask Isadora* (Masquerade Books) and *Let's Talk Sex* (The Crossing Press). Her first novel, *Bluebirds of Impossible Paradises*, will be published in 2001, and, of course it has lots of sex in it!

The online Sexuality Forum still flourishes at *www.askisadora.com*, and Isadora invites your questions and comments therein.

To Our Readers

Conari Press publishes books on topics ranging from spirituality, personal growth, and relationships to women's issues, parenting, and social issues. Our mission is to publish quality books that will make a difference in people's lives—how we feel about ourselves and how we relate to one another. We value integrity, compassion, and receptivity, both in the books we publish and in the way we do business.

As a member of the community, we sponsor the Random Acts of Kindness™ Foundation, the guiding force behind Random Acts of Kindness™ Week. We donate our damaged books to nonprofit organizations, dedicate a portion of our proceeds from certain books to charitable causes, and continually look for new ways to use natural resources as wisely as possible.

Our readers are our most important resource, and we value your input, suggestions, and ideas about what you would like to see published. Please feel free to contact us, to request our latest book catalog, or to be added to our mailing list.

2550 Ninth Street, Suite 101

Berkeley, California 94710-2551

800-685-9595 • 510-649-7175

fax: 510-649-7190 • e-mail: conari@conari.com

www.conari.com